Waiting is the Night

FINDING HOPE WHEN YOU'RE STUCK
ON THE OTHER SIDE OF DAWN

Waiting is the Night

SHANNON BRINK

AMBASSADOR INTERNATIONAL
GREENVILLE, SOUTH CAROLINA & BELFAST, NORTHERN IRELAND
www.ambassador-international.com

Waiting is the Night

Finding Hope When You're Stuck on the Other Side of Dawn

ISBN: 978-1-64960-594-8, hardcover
ISBN: 978-1-64960-375-3, paperback
eISBN: 978-1-64960-372-2

Cover Design by Hannah Linder Designs
Interior Typesetting by Dentelle Design
Edited by Marissa Earl

AMBASSADOR INTERNATIONAL
Emerald House
411 University Ridge, Suite B14
Greenville, SC 29601
United States
www.ambassador-international.com

AMBASSADOR BOOKS
The Mount
2 Woodstock Link
Belfast, BT6 8DD
Northern Ireland, United Kingdom
www.ambassadormedia.co.uk

The colophon is a trademark of Ambassador, a Christian publishing company.

I dedicate this book to my ever-loving and serving husband, Jason, who has cheered me on in every step of this journey (and helped me with too many technical things to keep track of). To my children who have brought more joy to me than I deserve. To my loving parents, stepparent, and in-laws for their continuous encouragement. To my mentors Janet Thiessen and Claudia Peterson for reading my writing, coaching my leading, and keeping me faithful. I am thankful to so many who have given me encouragement at each step to keep writing and giving me the confidence to share this piece of my soul in printed format.

Contents

Author's Note

I wish we could get a cup of coffee, you and I. The strong kind. The kind that can handle the tears we'd share. We have journeys that are painful, filled with waiting and grieving but also with joy. We are not so different. Maybe we are in different countries or longing for different things, but I know we would connect. I hope and pray that this book meets you where you need to be met the most. I encourage you to buy a new journal and a new pen, to sit with this book in a space where you can be free, and to truly reflect as you go. May God grant you your heart's desires; but even if He doesn't, may He meet you with more of Himself while you wait on Him. I suspect that He might be more than you ever hoped for.

Introduction

It is He who reveals the profound and hidden things;
He knows what is in the darkness, And the light dwells with Him.

Daniel 2:22

I am a creature of the night. Not by choice.

The dead of night and I have been at war for ten long years. The fear of the night has gripped me. Anxious and restless, sleepless and fearful, I repeatedly face clinical insomnia. In the dark of night when sleep eludes me, all I have left are endless thoughts that whirl and spin and flail. I wander dark hallways, trying to pass the time while my children and husband sleep. I look out windows to see shadowy streets and check the clock again and again. It is lonely being the only one awake.

There is something strange about living in the night. Corners and lines blur into smudges and shapes. The darkness can take on character and heighten emotions in ways that nothing in the daytime does. The air seems heavier somehow. The shadows seem fiercer and more oppressive. Time ticks by slowly and painfully.

Before these years of sleepless nights, I was not unfamiliar with roaming empty hallways and watching others sleep. Being a shift-working nurse required me to force my body beyond normal rhythms, carefully watching bodies and monitors as patients slept. Sometimes, with adrenaline surging through my veins, I would call Code Blues, prime intravenous tubing, and check pulses. But even in dark hospital corridors, while watching chests rise and fall under the dim lights, the night crawls by endlessly.

I was born on the West Coast of Canada, where the forests are dense with evergreens and moss-covered underbrush. As a child, camping in the forest was magical and ethereal. We imagined that the forest was a different world. But once you take away the light of day, the forest is no longer playful. It becomes foreboding and dangerous.

Branches become arms reaching out to grab those passing by; underbrush becomes monsters and creatures ready to pounce. I remember dreading any interaction with the forest by night. I would do anything to stay in my bed rather than get up to use the bathroom because the darkness would swallow me whole with fear and uncertainty.

In the middle of the night, there are no colors to be seen. There are only gray and black and shadow. There is little certainty of what things look like without the warm glow of daytime. In the middle of the night, it is hard to detect when dawn might arrive in blazing orange and purple hues. It can be disorienting. With time dragging and hope waning, it can feel like a lifetime.

For most people, night creates an atmosphere of rest and quiet, soul and body refreshment. But for one struggling to sleep, the night can become a wearying place with little reprieve. Struggling with insomnia is not something I wished for nor could have ever predicted. I used to run into bedtime like a freight train and pass out as soon as my head hit the pillow. Then in my mid-twenties, peaceful sleep turned into a place of restlessness and anxiety as a physical condition thrust me into sudden, perpetual insomnia.

Dawn never seemed to come for me. All I knew was the dark in-between of night. All I saw was the lingering black—never the glow of early sunrise.

Waiting is the Night

I can't help but think of the night when I think about waiting—for me, the two have become synonymous. My sleepless body inhabits the darkness of the night, but the darkness of night also inhabits me. I have spent more than my share of nights waiting for dawn to come. Waiting for time to pass. Waiting for a glimmer, a trickle of light to bounce off my walls. Waiting to hear soft noises of people and street sounds, anything to help me feel not so alone. In the ambiguous dark of night, the longing is almost palpable, for clarity is found only in the light of morning.

There is hope for the insomniac in that dawn does come. It must come; it will come. Nothing hinders dawn. Persistently, it comes. Predictably, it illuminates. There is no fear of a perpetual night. Maybe there will be no sleep, but there will always be light beckoning a new day.

The waiting soul, on the other hand, isn't always granted a definitive dawn. It might long for reprieve, for the realization of desires fulfilled and hopes restored. But as the waiting soul looks—as I have looked—to the horizon for something that it does not now have, will it receive what it longs for? What if the dawn never comes? What if the dark night remains? There is a hiddenness in waiting—a brokenness, a fearfulness, a weariness—as you watch out the window hoping for a bit of light, only to see your face reflecting back at you with its shadowy features ever unchanged.

For that soul, I have written this book. For that soul, I offer companionship, unchanging truths, and hope. For that soul, I say, *you are not alone.* Don't listen to the lie that claims you are alone as you wait on God in the thick of the night.

You who are trying desperately not to grow bitter as you look around at all those people in the glory of morning, all rested and shiny and bright. You who are confused, sitting in your dark night and wondering if you've been forgotten because God doesn't seem to be answering the desire of your heart even after so many years of longing. You who are so weary of unanswered prayers that you have lost all words to express them anymore. I will walk with you.

Whether you have lost hope or are clinging to your last few slivers of it, let's journey together in the night of waiting and look for the dawn. Maybe the dawn coming for you will not look like you think it will, but I believe it will come for you.

Blind Dining

For a new culinary experience, my husband and I once took friends of ours to Dark Table, a restaurant in Vancouver, Canada. Inspired by Jorge Spielmann, a Swiss man who blindfolded his guests in an attempt to show them what eating was like for a blind person, the entire eating experience is done in complete and utter darkness. There are no cell phones allowed, no windows, no light to be seen under door cracks.

Created to heighten the sense of taste while other senses are dulled, the restaurant also creates the beginnings of awareness for a person with sight of what living with total blindness is like. This amazing idea of blind dining also adds employment options for individuals with limited vision and, in a grand reversal, invites sighted people to be dependent on and led by those who are blind.

The immersive meal was unlike anything I have ever experienced. At first, it was so disorienting that I did not know how to behave properly. How loud was I supposed to talk? Did I open my eyes or leave them closed? I felt like my head was spinning in circles as my eyes drifted every which way, desperate to find some point of light with which to orient myself. But of course, there was none.

At first, it created such a panic in me that I started laughing inappropriately out of sheer nervousness and confusion. It was hard to settle in at the table or have meaningful conversation as the meal unfolded because I had to quiet my dominant, extroverted sense of sight in order to give way for my bashful and more introverted senses, like touch and smell.

In that situation, I recognized how much I rely on my sight for all the basic functions of life. How do I find my food on my plate if I cannot see it? How do I butter my bread? How do I walk through the restaurant to find the bathroom? When the server says, "Here is your plate of food" and I reach up, how do I find it? How do I know what I am even eating?

I do not pretend to imagine what it is like to be blind. Of course, a sighted person having a two-hour meal in the dark is nothing like the reality of blindness. But this eye-opening meal helped me understand my experiences with the darkness of my insomnia and helps now as I navigate a different kind of darkness—that of waiting.

When thrust into the world of darkness, I scrambled to find some bearing. Suddenly, what I thought I knew, I had to relearn. Edges of tables, what is up or down, what is near or far—everything became black, and it is was hard to maneuver. I became someone different in the dark. Where once I was so certain of every step and movement, I was now timid, worried, careful, slow, and unsure.

When we are in the dark times of our lives, when we have no clarity, we may act not too differently. There is a panic that rises when we are unable to depend on sight. We go from a place of seeing and knowing to blindness and uncertainty. How do we proceed when we feel clumsy and awkward? Even when it seems there is not a glimmer of light in our circumstances, as in the blind-dining experience, we're still given choices that help us navigate in the dark. We trust in the Server, Whose relationship to us is never uncertain. We hold confidence in unchanging truths that anchor us even in chaos: God will never abandon us in the darkness; His presence is always near to us; and we can trust in His ability to see what we would hardly even imagine.

When we cannot see, it becomes painfully obvious that we cannot rely on ourselves. We need God's nearness like never before. We have to slow down, call out, and grab hold of Him in ways we would never have had to if we always walked in the clarity of light. Huddled together, hands on shoulders at the Dark Table, we needed to put all of our trust in our server to guide us, calamity-free, through the restaurant and to our table. Like a line of children, we had to hold on to each other so that we wouldn't bump into anything. To let go of our server would have been futile.

So it is as we wait on God. It is in these times, when we cannot see, that we need His hand to guide; need to listen closely to His voice; need to settle into our unseeing, humble limitations; and allow ourselves to be led through the dark mystery before us.

What Are You Waiting For?

My entire work environment is a waiting room. In emergency rooms, I see the hollowed eyes, the twitching fingers, the clock glances from strangers and friends. In life, we are all alike in that we are all waiting alongside one another. We wait for painful seasons to pass. We wait for grief to stop gripping every waking moment. We wait for physical healing, for wayward children to come home, for babies to fill our empty wombs. We wait for the fruition of dreams, for callings, to be brought home, and to be sent out. We wait for justice, and we wait for oppression to end. Friends, we wait for so many things in this life.

Waiting is like the punctuation of creation: start, stop, wait, go again, and repeat. Light and dark rhythmically cycle after each other as day gives way to night, which turns back to day, and so on.

On Canada's West Coast, colors burst onto the scene in spring but only after the dark grays and blacks of cold winters. Animals emerge from hibernation; ice thaws; heat expands; leaves grow; and then everything contracts once more. Our own life mimics this pattern. We will have seasons of dawn and brightness, followed all too quickly by seasons of engulfing night.

All of us are waiting right now for something. Whether it's an unvoiced prayer, a silent urging, or a list of hopes and dreams, we are waiting. God's Word is bulging with stories of people who waited on Him just like us. All of humanity must wait for Him to come through, to answer, heal, provide, act on our behalf, guide, call, lead, and rescue.

Maybe the waiting isn't a surprise to you, but maybe the timing is. When it lingers well beyond when we thought it might, we can feel like every ounce of our patience has been wrung out and we are dry as a bone. Perhaps we were patient in the beginning, but now we are past our ability to go on. How do we reconcile ourselves to the idea that we might not even get what we are waiting for? What then?

What are you waiting for?

We often have very little control over our seasons of darkness. We are thrust into them without prediction or choice. We know that we will experience many and varied trials in this lifetime. We might have already endured hardships so painful that we cannot imagine why we would now find ourselves waiting for God's hand in something else. There is something altogether unique about the trial of waiting, versus other trials we face in this life. But what isn't unique is the truth that even when we do not choose the waiting, we choose our responses in the waiting.

Dawn

We love stories about the arrival of dawn, don't we? We love hearing about when a long-suffering night dweller finally gets to see the light of morning. We love the happy endings and the beautiful tying up of loose ends, and we inevitably gloss over the waiting years. Somehow, we focus on the light at the end of the tunnel, and we forget the darkness and disorientation that came before that light.

In longing for the other side, we sometimes relinquish the journey to get there. But we must remember, the Promised Land came only after the forty years in the desert. The filled womb came only after the longing of the empty one. We gloss over the waiting for a redeemer that took four hundred years. For us who wait, will there be an end to our waiting? If so, how long, O Lord, must we wait before what we most desire arrives? What do we do while we wait upon You?

God created the light to overcome the night. We know He can bring forth light from any darkness and sweep away all the pain of waiting with one swift answer. But do we know this even *while* we wait? Even while the night still looms heavy and endless in front of us? Before we know what the outcome will be? Before we see any change at all?

So then, how are we going to navigate in the dark?

In this book, I hope to lay before you truths about our choices in the night. Lurking in the shadows are lies and temptations that we might stumble upon and then cling to as we grope around. There are so many stories in Scripture which warn us of the common footpaths our souls can wander onto in our dark waiting rooms. These footpaths can lead us to shattered faith, despair, and bitterness. But there are also flickers of light in the dark nights which, if we hold out for them, will guide us instead toward a pathway of maturity and submission.

I believe that there will be a Dawn for you even as you wait, and His name is Jesus. He said, as recorded in John 8:12, "'I am the Light of the world; the one who follows Me will not walk in the darkness, but will have the Light of life.'"

I am journeying with you. Not as a dawn dweller, but as a creature of the night. I will be painfully honest about some of my own struggles and journeys as I, too, am in the dark waiting for God. Can we learn to be at peace with the waiting that may continue to define our circumstances? I am writing from a place of darkness in my candlelit corner, huddled under a blanket and watching the clock tick.

I am not writing from the bold, brilliant, white light of dawn. I am waiting upon God to do miraculous things in my own life but instead find myself learning about Him. I am waiting on God to bring something about, and yet He is bringing me about-face. I am waiting upon God to tell me how much longer *I* will have to wait. But He is reminding me of how long *He* is willing to wait for me to trust Him fully. I have asked for things, but He gives me more of *Himself.*

So here at this intersection, where we meet in the dark, let us journey together, arms linked like children, holding on to our Guide. Let us call out to Him for hope and wisdom to endure. Let us choose together to trust that He will indeed answer as we walk upon this path, knowing that though the horizon may yet be dim, the sun is still rising.

PART 1
The Way of the Flesh

"Come, let's return to the LORD.

For He has torn us, but He will heal us;

He has wounded us, but He will bandage us.

So let's learn, let's press on to know the LORD.

His appearance is as sure as the dawn;

And He will come to us like the rain,

As the spring rain waters the earth."

Hosea 6:1, 3

In the Dirt

Though born on Canada's West Coast, my family is currently serving as missionaries in East Africa. Living in the dirt here is a messy business. In this sun-soaked land which we now call home, dirt clings to and stains everything orange, including little feet and white school uniforms.

I used to love dirt, living on the Pacific coast of Canada. I spent hours with my hands in it, trying to make plants thrive and take root in locations around my yard. I displaced and relocated; I hovered and babied; I trimmed and fertilized. I hadn't a clue what I was doing, but I was determined to bring beauty and life.

I would spend hours hauling my children through nurseries on wet, soggy afternoons, dreaming of where to put each little life I brought home in its green pot. The only problem with my dream of possessing a beautiful garden is that I didn't realize how much death and loss went into a garden to make it thrive. I ended up endlessly frustrated. With one thriving plant came the death of another; with one wilting bush came a thriving weed. Aside from the work of planning and designing and holding back the forces of decay and death, most of my gardening ended up being about waiting.

So much waiting. Waiting to see if that plant would take. Waiting to see if the seeds would sprout. Waiting for another season for the plant to be fuller, better. Waiting for rain. Amending the soil. Picking out rocks by hand. Pulling weeds. Waiting to see if that plant would bloom this year. Waiting for beauty to erupt from the ground. Waiting months, seasons, and years.

I am in a season of life right now where I feel like all I am doing is waiting. Dreams and desires grip me, but it's not the right season. Hopes and visions rise in me, but then the weeds tug them down. I have been more than ready to throw down my shovel and give up on the work of gardening, and spiritually, I have done the same. Instead of being in awe of the comings-and-goings of seasons in my life, I run around like my gardening self—frantically trying to keep the beauty flourishing while holding off death.

I want the big reveal. I want God to bring about all my long-awaited hopes right now. I want everything in my life—all my hoping, all my being, and all my doing—to come together in some perfect symphony to create the full garden life. But it turns out, there seem to always be things for which I am waiting.

As with gardening, life isn't like I thought it would be. It's not about the things I thought it was about in my teenaged years. Life continues to lead me into places of greater tension. Even now, I am losing, and I am gaining. I am losing myself to my children and gaining myself back as my children need me less. I am expanding and contracting as my world around me does. Things I long hoped for have come to be, and other things I yet long for. Each season I live in has joys and sorrows. I wonder when the beauty of my incomplete life will capture me the way a garden full of life and death does. When will I be satisfied with all the loose, frayed ends and all the neat knots woven around the very heart of me?

The Light

The power outages we experience in our adopted country can be unsettling. They happen suddenly—when you have that pot on the stove, or you are trying to do homework, or you are just getting kids settled into bed. It's difficult to navigate without some source of light. Fumbling around in the dark is time-consuming and confusing. It makes you feel like a toddler, all awkward and prone to injury.

With every trial we face, we have a choice about how we walk. Our natural response when we have been thrust into the dark is almost immediately to make the darkness end. We run around trying to find the light switch, find a flashlight, and bring back the light. Darkness is scary, and nothing makes sense anymore. But when it turns out we have no control over the darkness, like our power outages, we then start trying to continue on as we always did, only in the dark. It's problematic. What we think we see, we misunderstand and misconstrue. Our behavior becomes erratic and, at times, idiotic, all because of the fear of falling or bumping into things. Pressing forward to find our own solutions, our own ways of managing, can lead to additional pain.

Unfortunately for us, the way of the flesh—to just keep going at the same pace and in the same direction, even though it is pitch black—is our natural tendency. We think we can navigate this trial of waiting our own way, without a guide. But it's like walking in the dark without a light. Unassisted by the light of Christ, we will walk straight into many obstacles, like difficult emotions, alluring temptations, and dangerous lies.

Is there another way? Instead of running around trying to find the light, trying to understand the dark on our own, or moving forward in our own wisdom, what might it look like to pause and lean into the dark? The way of the Spirit is a posture of trust, trusting that the dark is not purposeless, that He has something for us in it, and that we can navigate through it by His light to His glory.

There are many temptations as we fumble in the dark and wait for the things we desire—temptations to grab hold of things we think can help us, like a wobbly bookshelf or what we think is a stable handhold, temptations to let that "thing" we are waiting for guide us. Only then we find we have wandered toward a place we don't want to be. But if we let God guide us, we will not be overcome. Let us examine these temptations, test them, and see how to avoid them. Let us pause in the dark, take a deep breath, and call out for the light that only God's presence can give.

I know you are weary; I am, too. I know you are prone to wander; I am, too. But God's Word is filled to the brim with examples of other wanderers like us who had choices to make in their seasons of waiting on God in their seasons of darkness. Let us press on then, toward the prize (Phil. 3:14). Waiting is an inevitable reality of life on this side of Heaven and can be holy ground. God has more for us in seasons of waiting than we realize if we choose to walk in step with Him through our affliction.

CHAPTER ONE

What About My Good?

What shall we say then? There is no injustice with God, is there? Far from it! For He says to Moses, "I will have mercy on whomever I have mercy, and I will show compassion to whomever I show compassion." So then, it does not depend on the person who wants it nor the one who runs, but on God who has mercy.

Romans 9:14-16

There are many temptations in the land of waiting. Where will I rest my spirit, my thoughts, my heart when my dreams are on an altar ablaze? Will I rest my hopes and thoughts on God's goodness toward me, or will I focus on all that He seems to be keeping from me?

In a world of almost constant interruption and comparison, saturated with social media, it is so easy to let the whisper of envy invade the soul. It starts as a spark, a thought, a glance at a friend's social media. Then with very little work, it becomes a blazing, raging fire that consumes from the inside out. And I mean *consumes* us. It can be as insidious as a riptide, pulling slowly below our knees until, before we know it, our whole selves are swept out into the deep.

Temptation 1—Envy

Okay, so you are waiting for something, and it's hard—bone-wearying hard. Just like me waiting for healing from insomnia, it is crushing. But you don't wait in isolation. Herein lies the real challenge of waiting. You might be waiting, but maybe others are no longer waiting or have not waited at all. Perhaps those closest to you are living the dream that you want to live. They had another baby, while you still wait for yours. They bought that home. They got that dream job. They got to do what it is that you most long for in your heart. Echoing in response to this is the ache of your own heart, throbbing, "It's not fair!"

I've been reflecting on the story of Joseph and his family. My husband comes from a big family. There isn't much room in a large family for the spotlight to be on one person. Every decision requires lots of cooperating and group decision-making. So much so that the married-ins have often joked about the reality of his family's slow process. When everyone has to be considered, one person doesn't get the limelight, nor do they get to pursue their own personal desires at the expense of the larger group.

I kind of understand from where Joseph's brothers were coming. How did Joseph get to be the favorite? Of course, we know it is because he came from Jacob's favorite wife, but did they understand this? We know that he was handsome. Was that it? We know that he was smart and a quick learner. Perhaps he was a prideful brat, or maybe he was always rubbing his successes in his brothers' noses?

Having small children, I don't need an imagination to conjure what kind of sibling bragging and comparisons were happening in Joseph's home. How easy it would have been for them to envy him, to wonder at all the special benefits he got. How easy that dislike would have turned to outright hatred. I can only imagine how that must have brewed and festered. Their envy must have eaten away slowly at their contented hearts until it had stolen their security and confidence.

The fact that they all conspired to kill Joseph reveals the ultimate outcome of any envy, doesn't it? Envy leads to violence and broken relationships. Are we really surprised when the anger in their hearts turned to action? Their envy and hatred grew so significant that they considered killing their brother (Gen. 37:20).

My thoughts rage with doubts, among theirs. "Why did God give Joseph a dream, and not us? Does He still have a plan for us? Why does Joseph get special treatment? Has God forgotten us?" How quickly we look at another person's reality and judge our own. Joseph was given a dream, and instead of thanking God for His good gift, the brothers immediately compare it to their own stories. *But why not me?*

The truly miraculous thing is that God was working for their good *through* Joseph. God eventually provided for their rescue—saved them from death by starvation—through Joseph. Joseph would be a foreshadowing of Christ and the fact that although we hated Him, although we crucified Him, He was here to save us. How interesting I find this. It can be hard to believe that, in fact, God is working for our good in ways we cannot see. I often do not see the whole picture, so I envy others and how things seem to be "working out" for them, not realizing that God is always working things out for the good of all His people, including me.[1] I may not understand that "good," and it may not be defined in the same way that the world defines it, but God's Word assures me that His ways are not my ways.

Do I believe that God is really always working for the good of all His people and for His glory—even if it isn't in the way I thought He might? I cannot even imagine all the ways God will use the hard and turn even evil things to conform to His gloriously good plan. Did Joseph's brothers know that they were going to try to kill the very person whom God was planning to use to save them?

Envy is the most prominent thief of joy and community in my life. I speak from a recent and painful experience with this. I'll admit, I've circled the drain on this one as of late. I'm not writing from a place of conquering victory, but a place of weakness and brokenness.

1 Romans 8:28

I had a dear friend—a very dear friend. We whispered dreams together on walks and shared our hearts and our homes. We had very similar dreams that we believed were God-given, and we were both waiting and watching for God to fulfill them. We were taking steps of faith. We were each filling out applications. We were on our own journeys. And in the same season that God blew all her windows and doors open, He firmly shut mine.

Everything in me was so wounded, so grieved, so shocked by this abrupt change of plans that I could not seem to rally behind my friend, whose dreams were coming true. So, I distanced myself. Every time her name came up, I pushed away. I didn't celebrate. I didn't rejoice for her; I cried for me. I wanted to protect myself from the pain, but every interaction was about her sweet destiny, and all I could taste was bitterness in my throat. At the sheer mention of anything in her story, I was ripped apart.

I'm only now realizing how long envy has been my heart's natural inclination. Looking back, in so many seasons of my life, envy has been there calling me, prodding me, motivating me, defeating me. In this most recent season, all I could think was, *Why her? Why not me?*

Oh, I showed up; I pretended, and I went through the motions. But in my heart, I was firing daggers at her, and the truth is, I was saturated with envy. If you had pricked my heart, you would have seen only envy dripping out. It affected all my relationships and especially my relationship with this dear friend. It wasn't until a few weeks before she moved away that God hit me with the truth of my behavior. I had missed months with my closest friend. I had missed out because I was too focused on my own grief to rally behind her.

I've been wrestling over that experience in the last number of months. I justified my behavior because I was trying to protect myself. *It is too painful,* I told myself. *For my own sake, I had to walk away before I became bitter.* But was it time I needed? Was it space? Or did I actually need to confess my sin of unbelief in God's goodness toward me? I needed a healed heart from my envy and comparison and a renewed anchoring of my heart on the truth of

Scripture that God is for my good, too. How do we allow God to heal us while we are waiting, instead of accusing or withdrawing from others who are not waiting for the same things we are?

Well, I'd be lying if I said I had this all figured out. I don't. But one thing I've come to realize is the source of this envy in me. You see, it's a symptom, not the diagnosis. Envy comes from beliefs. It comes from the posture of my heart. I have been believing a lie that God is purposely withholding good from me. Where did I get that idea?

As the song by Chris Tomlin says, God is a good Father.[2] We cannot fathom the goodness of our loving, heavenly Father toward us—that He is always and forever for our good. So much so, that even things that are not good become reshaped and refashioned to become for our good.

The country we live in now does not recycle. Everything is thrown away as trash. There is trash everywhere; cardboard and glass and metal bits and bobs fill ditches and line the streets. It's hard to imagine that any of the plastic overflow could become something repurposed and lovely, but there are some artists and revisionists doing just that.

Plastic bottles are melted and twisted into fashionable earrings. Plastic bags are twisted, bent, and knotted to become handbags. Bottle caps are pounded and wrapped in cloth to make hot pads. It's miraculous and beautiful and incredible that the very rejected things become treasured things.

So it is with God: no part of our story is left without repurposing, no part thrown away as trash and neglected. He is using even the ugly and broken parts of our lives to reshape our characters. What seem like the worst parts become part of a greater story of beauty in the end.

Jesus asked, "Now which one of you fathers will his son ask for a fish, and instead of a fish, he will give him a snake?" (Luke 11:11). While I am asking God for things, waiting on His answers, He is working on my unbelief. I am having to learn to trust, and trust again, that God might not only know what

---

is best for me but actually does give me exactly what I need to fill me and fulfill His purposes through me in His timing and way.

The Lie—God Is Withholding Something Good

For the Lord God is a sun and shield; The LORD gives grace and glory;
He withholds no good thing from those who walk with integrity.

Psalm 84:11

Like a tsunami, motherhood swept in and almost swept me out to sea. I knew nothing of the deep waters of parenting. I didn't know my body would buckle and thrash and rail against all of the demands made of it. As every part of me was thrown around in the tumultuous waves, I barely kept my head above water. I focused on surviving for so many years that I didn't know how to enjoy the time, let alone savor it. Then six years in, God gave me the gift of a fourth child.

In the struggle to bring forth my first three children, I felt I had lost much of myself. Yet from within the bitterness of this loss, God gave me a sweet, new beginning. We named her Naomi, meaning "my delight." While I was enjoying all the little moments with her as a baby, God was reclaiming and redeeming the early years of mothering when I just couldn't see past my own pain.

I delight in Naomi so much that sometimes I can barely breathe. But it begs a bigger question: Do I believe God delights in me in the same way? Do I believe He delights in me and withholds nothing good from me for the sake of my joy and His glory? Can it be that He loves me like that?

If I dig deep enough, under the pungent aroma of my envy, I find a root that goes deep down: I don't really believe that God is for my good. I don't really believe that He truly delights in me and will stop at nothing to bring about good plans for me out of the fullness of His unrelenting love—because I think I know what those good plans should be.

On the surface, we want so many things, so many dreams, that when we don't have those things, we start to think He's withholding them from us. But we are, as my little delight is, His joy. It's only the enemy who lies to us to tell us otherwise.

This lie cuts to the heart of us, but of course, it's a very old lie. In fact, it is a tattered, worn, and frayed lie that the enemy has been dragging around like my daughter drags her baby blanket. He has been using it since the very beginning of humankind. Satan convinced Eve that God was withholding the good fruit from her. He said that once Eve ate the fruit, she would get an amazing ability to be like God. Therefore, God forbidding her to eat it was Him withholding something good. Of course, we know that those limits were there to protect Adam and Eve, not prevent them from good.

How is it that Satan still tricks me with this one? When I consider the posture of my heart, it's almost like I think God owes me good things as *I* define them like prosperity, purpose, pain-free living, explanations and reasons.

God doesn't owe me the things I want, but out of His love, He gives me all the good I *need*, as He defines them. I am a created being. I cannot determine my own next breath. I am like "dust" and "a vapor" (James 4:14).

I find it horribly hard to read the end of the book of Job. I have walked shoulder to shoulder with Job until his shadow has rubbed a permanent indentation in my side. I know him well. I get him in ways I hoped I'd never understand. His life was robbed of so many good things. Children, flocks, prosperity, health—all the things for which we long. Yet at the end of all of the ruminating and questioning and wondering with his friends about his circumstances, after they've given many answers from the human book of understanding for why all of this awful stuff has been happening to Job, how does God finally respond to Job? Does He give a paltry explanation? A nimble excuse? God doesn't actually explain anything to Job about his circumstances. It's maddening, really.

God doesn't give Job a reason why at all. Instead, God answers Job with so much evidence from creation—evidence that piles up and spills out over everything in a deep layer—that it proves beyond any doubt that God is Sovereign and withholds no good thing. He rules over all, and His ways cannot be thwarted, nor do they need to be defended to us, His mere creation.

I have long pondered this absence of an explanation to Job and have found a piercingly simple possibility. It was illustrated when my husband and I were watching a movie recently, one in which the main character is put on trial for being a spy. Throughout the whole movie, the lead is seen as practically expressionless. He appears to be unmoved by the fact that his life is on the line. So many times, his lawyer asks him, "Aren't you worried? Aren't you concerned?" and every other variance on this question. But this man's response was eye-opening to me. He simply says each time, "Would it help?" That is the real question.

Would it help if I knew why I am facing the waiting, the trials, the afflictions that I am facing? Would any answer really comfort me? Or do I need to simply hold on to the truth that God is good and withholds no good thing from me?

For a few years, I worked in a pediatric emergency room. I've seen any number of children in severe pain, often at the hands of healthcare workers. Of course, we are not trying to do harm. We are doing good, but healing often begins by having to do something a bit painful. Have you ever tried to insert a tiny IV into barely visible, two-year-old veins? It involves holding arms down, tying tight bands around little limbs, squeezing hands, pinching with a needle, and advancing tubes into veins. It hurts! Despite all we do to explain and reduce the pain, the reality is that it hurts, and no real explanation to little children helps remove their hurt. Does explaining to a two-year-old that they need intravenous antibiotics to fight off their sepsis so that they can live for the next eighty years help them be more able to endure the pain? Not really!

So it is with me—I am that two-year-old. I cannot fully see what God sees. Any small explanation would be insufficient to comfort Job. Any explanation would likely not have removed the immediate trauma Job was experiencing.

Thousands and perhaps millions of people's eyes have cried rivers over reading Job and finding comfort in the fact that they are not alone in their difficulties. How could God explain all the ways in which Job's story would be woven in with our stories and the riches of the comfort we would find within it? Could that be summarized, quantified, and laid out so that Job would say it was worth it?

In his moment of pain and heartache, I'm not sure it would have helped him. It certainly wouldn't have removed the current sting. Could it be that Job was not given an answer for our sake? If Job had been given one, wouldn't we also expect one in our own circumstances? Somehow it quiets my soul's questioning to see Job's unwavering faith even though He never found out why He was suffering.

God doesn't answer about Job's circumstances but instead puts Job on the stand. What does Job know, anyway? "Do you give the horse *his* might? Do you clothe his neck with a mane? Do you make him leap like locusts?" (Job 39:19-20). On and on God continues. I can almost see Job sinking smaller and smaller back into that speck of dust from where he began. Of course, Job can't answer because he does not know what God knows. The answer to all of God's questions is "I am a mere man." Our understanding, compared to His, is so ridiculously finite, it takes but one chapter of text—thirty verses exactly—to silence Job's lips and put him in his right place.

Who am I to judge what God is doing in my life? Who am I to doubt His goodness, His grace to me? Can I even fathom what He has prevented me from enduring, from all that He's saved me? Can I even grasp, but for a second, what He is working in me because of my waiting? Can you?

We are but human, finite, limited in our understanding. We do not understand the length of our own days. We are so completely and utterly small and helpless, yet our lack of trust implies that God is in our debt.

He owes us nothing but gives us everything. The Bible is clear that He gives us everything we need for life and godliness.[3] He is, Himself, our abundant life. But do we trust Him with all that we yearn for? Is He given the chance to be the answer to the "what" for which we're actually waiting?

For Further Reflection

1. Do you believe that God is working for your good? How have you seen Him working? Or do you believe that He is withholding from you? Why?

2. Reflect on God's timely provisions for you in the past. Meditate on all the ways He has already proven that He is, indeed, for you.

3. In what ways are you accusing God instead of trusting Him and accepting the comfort He is offering you?

---

3   2 Peter 1:3

CHAPTER TWO

Dreams and Plans

I certainly believed that I would see the goodness of the LORD

In the land of the living.

Wait for the LORD;

Be strong and let your heart take courage;

Yes, wait for the Lord.

Psalm 27:13-14

As I watch my growing boys scale East African trees like monkeys and speed down bumpy paths on bikes, I inwardly cringe. I know too much and have seen so much pain on little bodies that it is difficult to watch them conquer heights and obstacles with agility and speed while always imagining their fatal demise. I have not forgotten their baby skin and cannot stomach the idea that it now covers boy bodies and bulging personalities that believe in their own invincibility. But the tension remains—I cannot hold them close to me forever. I cannot protect them from everything, shielding them from the exhilaration of conquering their surroundings. I need to let go—but not yet completely.

Temptation 2—Giving Up on the Dream

Our lives are filled with tension. How tightly should we hold our hopes and dreams in our hands, while also loosely enough that God can easily pluck them from us if He asks? I think of a runner at the starting line, a sprinter at the top of her game. Her muscles are tense; she is holding her position. One leg is crouched beneath her, the other stretched long and lean behind her. Her foot is on the starting block, and she is ready. Oh, she is ready. She waits, tense, listening closely, steady in her position. She is unmoved, yet expectant, because she is prepared and ready for the gun to fire.

What would it look like to live like that? Expectant and believing that God has plans for us—plans to bless us, to expand His kingdom through us, and perhaps to fulfill the dreams He has placed in us. Might we be willing to wait at the starting block for the right time and the right way in which He might lead?

Yet it is so terribly tempting to walk away from the starting block. When the time takes too long, when things aren't happening as quickly or as perfectly as we hoped they might, we move our eyes from the finish line. We get off the block and wander away. We forget about the race we were called to run. We stop training and move away from the track. He is too long in coming; maybe our long-expected Savior is not on His way, after all. He is so long in coming that we forget to wait for Him at all. When there is no hope, we fade away, disillusioned, and stop believing in bigger things. Then when He does call us and says, "It's time," we are not ready.

Have we stopped expecting God to show up? Have we closed the chapter, shut the book, and stopped believing He can do great and mighty things in and through us or on our behalf in our waiting?

It is tempting, in the waiting, to abandon our dreams altogether. It's too painful to imagine that they might not come about in the way we hope, so it is easier to pretend we don't have them. Maybe we get busy elsewhere or follow another's dreams instead. We decide that something less is best. But maybe, just maybe, we're meant to wade into the depth of them, ready to see where God takes us.

As uncomfortable as it is, is it possible to sit in the discomfort a little bit longer? Is it possible to sit in the darkness with eyes wide open—in the wanting, the longing, the hoping for—without abandoning hope or abandoning God altogether? Do we trust that He will enter into our waiting with us and guide us along the path that He has planned for us all along?

I wonder sometimes if I don't wait long enough for Him to show up in order for Him to minister to me. I'm so uncomfortable not knowing what's ahead that I don't sit still long enough for Him to meet me there in the pain of my waiting. It hurts my eyes staring out in the dark for too long.

The Lie—God Does Not Have a Plan for Me

"For I know the plans that I have for you," declares the Lord . . .

Jeremiah 29:11

Noah was one who waited long for the fulfillment of a God-given vision. Maybe you are like Noah, in that God has given you a vision, a specific dream, a hope, or a calling, and you believe He will bring it about. In fact, His message to you was so clear it is indisputable (I envy you, by the way). But the problem is that it's not coming about nearly as fast as you thought it would come. In fact, the fulfillment of that dream is not even close to within your grasp.

It's tempting to doubt. It's tempting to let it go, but you keep moving forward. In fact, you feel like a fool. Everyone thinks you're crazy. You're starting to think you're crazy.

Well, you're in good company. I wonder how frustrated Noah became as he waited for the rains to come. He was certainly busy preparing for the flood and building an ark. The Bible is unclear on exactly how many years passed from when God told Noah to start building to when the flood arrived. But imagine the seasons passing, the clock ticking, lives ebbing and flowing throughout, perhaps, decades. What faith was required of Noah to continue sawing and cutting boards, hammering and constructing an ark, to endure such a long wait without falling into doubt and confusion! How quickly we lose heart and vision when God tells us something and doesn't do it right away.

But we do know that one of the reasons for such a long wait for Noah was God's mercy. God waited for the people of Noah's time to repent. He didn't flood the earth right away, but throughout the time that Noah was building, and even before, God waited and was long-suffering to provide grace. He waited to give that generation opportunity for salvation, but they did not take it. Noah was waiting, but so was God.

But we learn some things from Noah in his waiting—namely, obedience with the few small steps that God gave him without needing to know the big picture and how everything was going to happen. There was not a single act of obedience but instead, daily obedience—daily waking up and being present to the task at hand, to build more and more without proof of the flood coming. Maybe it would have been easier if things were changing in nature around him, if he heard newscasters talk about global warming or environmental shifts. But perhaps nothing changed. Everything stayed the same, except that Noah had faith that something was coming because God told him so.

I also find it interesting how little God told Noah about how things were going to happen. Or at least, Scripture doesn't tell us all the details. Noah was told specifications for the ark he was supposed to build,[4] whom he was going to take, and what supplies to include. He was told that he needed to take two of every animal. But what's interesting is what he was not told. He was not told precisely how long it would take to build the ark. He was not told how the animals would get on the ark. He was not told how long the flood would last or if it would recede at all. He didn't know if others would join him on the ark and likely had no frame of reference for what a flood would look or feel like.[5] But his faith was firm.

Noah didn't understand the big picture. He didn't understand that through him would come all the people on the earth after that point.

4   Genesis 6:15
5   Hebrews 11:7

He didn't know for certain that God would place his feet on solid earth again. God didn't even mention that. He was told only a few things at first, possibly forty-some years before the flood happened, and what did he do? "So Noah did *these things*; according to everything that God had commanded him" (Gen. 6:22).

How often we want to know a hundred steps from where we are. We want to see the road map. "I can wait for a while, as long as I know that the waiting will one day end, as long as I know I'll get what I want. The wait will be worth it if I know what's waiting on the other side." But it is indeed rare that God works like that, isn't it? Faith and trust require obedience one step at a time. In your waiting season, you don't know all that is ahead. You don't know when God will do what He has revealed to you. You don't know what it might look like on the other side. But what has He told you to do right now? What is your one step? I'm guessing He has told you enough to be obedient right now. I'm guessing you know enough to trust Him.

Maybe you are like Noah, and you have to ask yourself, "Can I wait for as long as it will take for God to do what He told me He would do?" Will you continue faithfully serving, faithfully waiting, faithfully trusting that God is Who He says He is and will do what He says He will do, in His perfect timing? Do you believe that He will reveal more to you when you need to know it, not before or after?

Sometimes, perhaps like myself, you feel like you have been obedient by putting the seeds in the dirt, and you stand there watching the earth for a hint, just a hint, that life will grow from your obedience. Eyes to the dirt, face to the wind, you water and watch and hope and pray, and still you wait for that little shoot of green to prove your obedience worthwhile. No act of obedience is unseen; it will produce fruit. Though it looks buried in the dirt, God is at work in that seed, doing the miraculous in places unseen. Can you believe a little longer?

For Further Reflection

1. What is your heart's desire? What have you told God about it?

2. How has God revealed some aspect of His desires for your life?

3. How do you need God to reassure you right now that He still has plans for you even as you wait for them to be revealed?

4. Is there a step you were supposed to take, but you didn't because the whole plan isn't clear? If so, what was it? What is the next step you could take right now that God has already told you?

CHAPTER THREE

Trusting the God of Miracles

Trust in the Lord with all your heart and do not lean on your own understanding.

Proverbs 3:5

Don't you just love how the Bible passes over not months but sometimes years of people's lives without giving you any details? They can end up resembling cardboard cut-out people, not emotional, desire-ridden, three-dimensional, flesh-covered people like us. But when you try their skin on for a while, when you really enter into their stories, it's not hard to imagine the noise of their internal dialogue.

Lately, all I can see in Scripture are the longing faces, impatient hearts, and frustrated timelines of the people filling its pages. After Noah, I don't have to search long for other waiting souls—Abram and Sarai. At the beginning of their story, God spoke so clearly to them, telling them exactly what was going to take place. He told them to get up, move to a new land, and have a family.[6] God's clear direction did not make the road easy, however.

Temptation 3—Making It Happen on Your Own

Abram was seventy years old when God told him and Sarai to get up and move and that their offspring would be innumerable as the stars.[7] They

---

6   Genesis 12:1-3
7   Genesis 15:5

believed and obeyed. Packing up their household and wandering over the lands, Abram and Sarai walked in faith. Or it seems like they did in those first years. I don't doubt that their hearts were bursting with the excitement and adventure that lay before them. I can hear their late-night conversations. "God has chosen us! He has big things in store!" I can only imagine their twinkling eyes and humble hearts and how exciting it would have been—for the first few years. God said He would make them into a great nation. Yet they wandered rootless, like nomads, until they finally settled in a place near Hebron. Then in the Bible passages that follow, after God's great vision was laid before them and they had packed up and moved their entire lives, they waited twenty-five years before they had any children to begin forming a "great nation."

Twenty. Five. Years.

Has anything similar happened to you? God reveals part of a picture to you, a glimpse of a vision, and you are ecstatic. You jump on board. You file the application for the adoption. You sign up with a missions agency. You quit your job and start your own business. You've decided to start a family. You hear from God; you start the journey; and you are excited. It's all really happening! There are fundraisers for your adoption. There is progress with your business. You are finally in the middle of "God's will." Then, nothing—or closed doors, or waiting for that child to come, or infertility, or financial difficulty, or nothing but moments fading into months, fading into years, as time passes and your dreams wither. At this point, the enemy of our souls is there, hovering in the wings as he has since the beginning, prodding us to question God's faithfulness.

Where was Sarai in all this? The story of her family continued; time passed, but I can imagine that her mind was often resting on the topic of her aching, empty womb. If she were anything like me, she was crying on her bed, again, wondering why in the world this was not happening as it was supposed to. If she'd had a pharmacy, how many trips would she have taken to buy pregnancy tests? How many times would she have tracked her monthly cycle only to be disappointed again? How many women did she watch grow with child, bear that baby, and then raise that child to become a teenager? How that longing would have grown and grown. Twenty-five years is a long time when you are waiting for a child.

Nothing much is said about Sarai's faith during this long season, but I would not be surprised if she was as dry as a desert inside. Tears were cried and prayers uttered until there were no more words. She probably had many conversations with Abram asking why God would move them around the globe but not fulfill His promise about offspring. I can only imagine how lonely this would have felt.

But then, like a glimmer of light on the horizon after a long and dark night, the sun came up. There was a fresh word from God. Imagine the sweet relief flooding their souls as God finally spoke again and encouraged, "'Now look toward the heavens and count the stars, if you are able to count them. . . . So shall your descendants be'" (Gen. 15:5). Like water on parched ground, how hope would have seeped in. Like a warm blanket on a cold night, how peace would have enveloped them.

I can almost lean in and hear Sarai's thoughts. There would have been worship. There would have been joy. There would have been excitement and peace again. "Our God has not forgotten us! We will have children! God spoke it; it will happen." In this incredible meeting with God, Abram was shown the heavens and told that as surely as the stars are innumerable in the sky, so would his children be.

If I were Sarai, I would have started buying baby clothes and, perhaps, examining my abdomen and concluding it was indeed swelling. I would have assumed that what God had said was as good as done, right then. I might have told a few people, prepped the nursery, and presumed to know exactly what God intended. We love to have a plan, don't we? Oh, how I enjoy details, specifics, dates on calendars, and tidy conclusions. Mystery is not inviting when it comes to life plans; I like certainty.

Of course, we learn that many more years would pass before Sarai would be pregnant with a child.[8] During those years, when it was hard to see an end to that waiting season, imagine the darkness that descended upon her. All she saw was the waiting, longing, and yearning—hopes which felt crushed under the weight of time. Her hopes may have dragged down like the sagging of her aging skin. Maybe she was supporting Abram all along and her faith was holding on by a thread, but with the death blow of another year, and another, she simply could not believe the impossible could happen. She started to doubt her role. Maybe God chose Abram, but He certainly hadn't chosen her. How could something miraculous come from a body that was aging by the day, from a body that had let her down for years? I doubt she had much hope at all.

Do you feel an inkling of anger on Sarai's part? I do. Perhaps bitterness? Despair? Just thinking of it makes me want to weep for her sake. Is it any wonder that in Genesis 16, we see Sarai trying to make things happen on her own? An unknown number of years after God's initial covenant, we read her groanings to Abram that "'the LORD has prevented me from bearing *children*'" (Gen. 16:2). That phrase is wrapped up in rejection and shame and disappointment, isn't it? As a woman, I know how we internalize the shame of our body's failings as our own. What was her self-worth like at this point?

I can imagine that if she had a mirror to stare into, if she saw sagging and wrinkled cheeks and paper-thin skin, she would have been disbelieving. Wouldn't you be? Was God cruel to dangle a long-felt desire and dream before their faces without any indication of when it was going to happen? With the reality of their infertility closing in on them as the years waned, who could hold on to hope? *It would be impossible now*, Sarai probably thought. *I mean, look at me.* Our bodies are a frequent reminder that time is passing and youth is indeed only a fleeting season. Maybe the clincher was that she had now not only entered menopause but had also passed through it. As months passed

---

without a cycle, she saw that her womb was closed—for good. All she could see was what the eyes of her flesh could see—impossibility.

So began Sarai's journey to fulfill God's vision on her own. Most of us will, at some point in our lives. We decide that we are simply going to go it our own way. God seems slow in keeping His promises, and we are running out of time. Sarai decided that since what God had spoken of was physically impossible, she would present to her husband her servant, Hagar, who would sleep with Abram and provide an heir for him. Somehow, she convinced Abram that this had to be the path to take.

That seems like a strange idea, doesn't it? It might seem odd to us now, but it wasn't so uncommon in Abram's time in the Near East to give servants over for the production of offspring. Aside from the strangeness of her solution (to us), the reality for Sarai was that her choice, to do the miraculous work of God without God, led to terrible consequences in her and her family's lives. It wasn't so much her actions as her lack of faith behind them.

Maybe Sarai had an advantage. After all, God spoke *aloud*, directly to Abram to promise an heir. However, looking back, maybe she thought, *He never clearly said whose womb would bear the offspring, did He?* Nonetheless, whether the point of which woman would bring forth the nations was clear to Abram and Sarai, it's not so hard to imagine that the ongoing waiting could have muddled their emotions. When things didn't go according to the plan or timeframe for which they hoped, how easy it might have been to assume that God wasn't going to follow through. I can't really blame her, can you? I see too much of myself in her. I so quickly see the limitations of my circumstances and doubt that God can work *in the midst of them*. I often think I need to get *out* of my circumstances for Him to work. Most of the time, I don't even look for His miraculous intervention anymore. I'm too busy planning my own plan B.

So, Hagar produced an heir, which caused strife and struggle and jealousy and pride and every other ugly, sinful behavior between the two women. I can't imagine the divide this also caused between Sarai and her husband. Knowing your servant slept with your husband, that she had a child, and then having her hold that over you? What did it feel like for Sarai to see Abram delight in his son, Ishmael, knowing she wasn't the mother? I imagine the bitterness that rose up in the back of her throat, the grief—or perhaps even the feelings of rejection and envy.

I am in the middle of a place in my own life where the temptation to "go my own way" awakes with me every morning. It seems to take every single power within me to refuse to walk the way Sarai did. This looks different in each situation. In my case, God said to wait for something I desire, but my own impatience with His timeline tempts me to try to push open doors He has clearly shut for now. What is it in me that so desires to move ahead on my own, even without God's direction?

For me, it starts with fear. *Maybe those desires weren't from God from the start. Maybe I heard Him wrong.* "Did God really say . . . ?" I have carried this nagging doubt with me from the time I was a child: "Maybe God picked everyone except me to do His work." The lies start popping up like weeds. I keep grabbing at them, trying to pull them out, but the roots go deep.

I imagine Sarai may have had her own weeds of self-doubt. I imagine she was exhausted from pulling them up and had just given in and given up.

In what ways do you see seeds of independence or fear rising up in you? Or are you so far down your road to plan B that you are not even sure you can go back to the beginning?

The thing is, at the end of Sarai's story, we see a miracle. Out of the ashes of the desolate solution she had planned, God renewed His covenant again when Abram was ninety-nine years old. And within a year, Isaac was born. Despite her sin, God's plans were not derailed. This miracle was not of her own doing. Nor was it deserved on her part. Their story, from a human perspective, had already ended. In fact, their story was shut, and its book was tucked away on a dusty, old shelf. Sarai and Abram could do nothing to produce offspring. They had no power; they had no ability to overcome the very real obstacles of age and infertility. When there was nothing else to be done but wait on God—to look to Him, hope in Him—it was then, and only then, that the miracle came. Not because of anything they had or hadn't done but because it was God's timing, and He was faithful to do what He had promised. Only, He got the glory, not them. There is no way they could have interpreted the provision of an heir as anything *but* God's doing. They could not work it up, work it out, or work through it. He did it.

Maybe it's the same for us. Without God showing up in our circumstances, in our stories, the miracles won't happen. That desire we hold, that person we want to become, that dream we want to see realized—maybe they are from Him, but their fruition is meant to be *by* Him and for His glory and fame, not ours.

The truth is, I kind of want the glory sometimes. I want the solution to be the result my effort and strength and doing. I act as though it all depends on me. Then when the outcome is what I desire, I can take claim to it. But it's God's story and His glory.

The Lie—God Cannot Really Do the Impossible

Is anything too difficult for the Lord?

Genesis 18:14

Something from nothing, a virgin's womb filled with a growing Savior, parting seas, water turned to wine, blinded eyes opened—our God is a God of the impossible. Our God is the God of miracles. To imagine that He can carve out stars from the void with just a word from His lips, that He can breathe into dust and make everlasting souls, displays a magnitude of greatness we cannot even conceive. Yet I so often doubt that in this chapter of my story, He can do something new, something unimaginable, something miraculous. Is it possible for Him to pull out pages, write with new ink, white out the lies, and start new things in my life? Do I believe it?

Ultimately, this temptation to do things on our own stems from disbelief that God can really do the impossible.

Why do I have such a hard time believing for miracles in my own life? Maybe it's because I doubt His choice. Maybe it's because I feel I am so saturated with sin that I soak everything around me with it, and I can't imagine He can work through me in such a state. I sometimes struggle to remember that God uses us despite our weaknesses and failings. What a miracle that He can work in any and all persons, in any and all circumstances, whether we feel we deserve Him using us or not. Maybe I just haven't waited for the sunrise long enough. Would I wait differently if I knew dawn was just a breath away? With bleary eyes, gasping yawns, and heavy exhaustion, can I keep my eyes open just long enough that I don't miss the miracle about to take place as day breaks forth?

Many of us are waiting for a desire to be fulfilled, and we cannot seem to shake those longings, hopes, and visions for our lives. We've asked God to fulfill the desire, to remove it, to do something about it; but still, we wait. We desperately want to be in a relationship; we desperately want to have children; we want to travel; or we want to find our "calling" and mission. We pray; we ask; we beg; we plead; and it seems like time is running out.

I think of another story in Scripture—that of Elizabeth and Zacharias in Luke 1. It is similar to the story of Abram and Sarai, as they, too, were longing for a child. But the difference between their stories is stark: while Sarai caused a series of events that nearly destroyed her family as she waited, Elizabeth and Zacharias remained faithful to the waiting. The New Testament couple also experienced firsthand the miraculous work of God, but they faithfully held out to see the glorious miracle arrive, without the repercussions of going their own way in the meantime.

I find it interesting how the Bible says Zacharias and Elizabeth were highly praised, highly regarded before the Lord, and that Zacharias served in the temple; but still, they were childless.[9] How quickly we presume that we

---

9 Luke 1:6–7

have done something wrong to deserve unfulfilled desires. How quickly we believe that God does not hear our prayers or see our longings. How quickly we doubt that He is the One Who gave us those desires.

In hindsight, we know that God was waiting for the perfect moment in history for John the Baptist to be conceived in Elizabeth's womb. We know now that there was more going on behind the scenes. We see that God planned to bless them beyond anything they imagined—with a child that would not only be remarkable in every way but would serve God from birth until death. John the Baptist prophesied and prepared the way for Jesus, the Savior of the world. But would Elizabeth and Zacharias have been able to raise John the way they needed? Would they have been able to steward God's calling on them if they had dissolved into bitterness about all that God was keeping from them?

Imagine the intermingling of hope and pain and long-suffering as Zacharias entered the temple to bring his prayers again to his Father—prayers for a Savior, for a Messiah, and for a son. And beauty was waiting just around the corner, converging all of their hopes and dreams into one answer: John, who prepared the way for Jesus. However, how might John have grown up if his parents were scarred with bitterness and resentfulness from their years of faithfully serving while their home and hearts and her womb remained empty? Would the outcome have been the same if they hadn't continued coming to God, waiting on Him, and asking of Him? Would Gabriel have appeared to Zacharias at all if he had stopped serving in the temple and they had abandoned all faith? But that didn't happen. God chooses whom He chooses, but nonetheless, we have a part to play by continually humbling ourselves to the mighty hand of God. I am so inspired that they stayed the course, continuing to serve and give, even though we can imagine how their hearts hurt.

While it might have been easy for Elizabeth and Zacharias to give up hope, what we see instead is their steadfast faithfulness. Zacharias continued to serve in the temple. They persisted in obeying and following God. They persevered in a march toward righteousness, even though it hurt that they did not have any offspring to call their own. Infertility is hard today in our own culture; how much harder it would have been in Jesus's time. Many might have assumed Zacharias and Elizabeth had done something horrible to deserve God's wrath,[10] such that God had afflicted Elizabeth to her own fault. They may have felt the disgrace or the disdain from other Jews around them. What a relief to find out from this story that God's favor isn't always proven in the short term but is sometimes proven in the long term. They waited on the Lord and served Him, even when their hearts were broken. That is a tall order—one which I struggle to follow.

Do you believe that God can still do the impossible in you in your circumstance? Do you believe He is still faithful, even when you cannot see? Your posture toward Him and your continued obedience to praise and serve Him, no matter what the outcome, will determine everything about what happens to your heart and character as you wait.

For Further Reflection

1. What long-standing dreams have you abandoned because God hasn't brought them about right away? What would it take for you to find those dreams and desires again, to not abandon them, but choose to wait upon the Lord?

2. Are you more like Sarai and Abram or Zacharias and Elizabeth? Why?

3. Do you believe God can still do miracles in your situation? Why or why not?

---

10 Luke 1:25

CHAPTER FOUR

The Hard-Hearted Quest for Fairness

Come, let's worship and bow down,

Let's kneel before the LORD our Maker.

For He is our God,

And we are the people of His pasture and the sheep of His hand.

Today, if you will hear His voice,

Do not harden your hearts.

Psalm 95:6-8

I sit here watching my kids etch in the Malawian dirt with a stick for hours. The dirt in the dry season is hard like stone. After months without rain and pancake-smooth, the ground seems impossibly indurated. Grinding their little stones and sticks into it, they cannot get beyond the tough-as-nails crust of the dirt. Even if they do, they find that beneath it is just another equally solid layer. They keep at it, determined to discover gold in our backyard. They scrape but get nowhere.

Temptation 4—Bitterness

I think bitterness is like this hard earth. Sun-scorched, weary, and set, no seeds can be sewn in hardened land. Not until it is softened and moistened and worked into by water, by tools, and by sweat. I think of my heart. I think of the difficult seasons I have gone through, dryness and heat evaporating hope and faith. Have I become this impenetrable soil, this destitute place that is hard in my God's hands?

When I think of a person who had ample opportunity to become bitter by life's circumstances, I think back on the story of Joseph and examine him thoroughly. He had every reason to become bitter at God, didn't he? He did not ask to be Jacob's favorite. He certainly did not ask to receive his brothers' deceit or to be cast away by them because of his dad's favoritism. He definitely did not deserve to be a slave in a foreign land, imprisoned by their demands. God gave Joseph a vision that he would have a position of authority and that his brothers would bow to him, yet he became a slave.[11] I would be bitter, wouldn't you? Yet we see that God was with him, that He showed favor to Joseph, and that He did not leave him alone. But like the earth, which is subject to weather and seasons and the whims of nature, Joseph's troubles were only beginning.

Joseph's life would be mocked and humiliated. He would be promoted only to be demoted; he would be falsely accused and imprisoned; and he would be cast away. But after years of this kind of treatment, Joseph did not ultimately use these circumstances as an excuse to sin. By God's mercy, we do not see him growing hard and bitter. He remained righteous though tempted with pride and greed and kept his head to the ground, working and waiting.

We don't know for certain the posture of Joseph's heart. We don't know if he tossed and turned in his sleep for years, trying to shed himself of the anger that no doubt could have enveloped his heart. We don't know if he played tug of war with God, asking, "Why me?" or "Why now?" or "How come?" his brothers had hated him to the point of abandonment. We don't find out any of this.

However, when the dust settled and God indeed put Joseph in a position of power and authority and allowed his brothers to lay prostrate before him as his vision had foreseen, we do not see Joseph bitter. We do not see him hard as stone, unforgiving, unrelenting, and unmerciful. Instead, we see a broken man. Joseph

---

11 Genesis 37

wept so loudly that the Egyptians wondered at his unabashed show of emotion. He wept and clung to his brothers, *forgiving* them even to the point of telling them not to be angry at themselves for their own sin and that God had not abandoned their family because of their sin. What they had intended as harm, God had used for His good.[12] What a declaration of faith! It is enormous and powerful in my own heart. At the end of all his affliction, after years of being cast aside and tossed about far from all he'd known and almost as a refugee in a foreign land, Joseph was tender. His heart was like soft dirt that crumbles in one's hand. Tender, malleable, and trusting his Father, not bitter and hard.

We have every opportunity to sin in our seasons of waiting. We have every reason, from a fleshly perspective, to rail against God. We can blame Him; we can be angry at Him; we can throw our fists in the air and demand that God change His way with us. Or we can humble ourselves and be reminded that "the fear of the LORD is the beginning of wisdom" (Prov. 9:10). We can lie flat on the earth and wait for the rain of His mercy. We can allow His presence to soften our hearts like clay in His hands, becoming malleable and tender. We can choose to submit, or we can choose to become bitter. One way leads to life; one way leads to death.

The Lie—God Is Unfair

Do you not know? Have you not heard?

Has it not been declared to you from the beginning?

Have you not understood from the foundations of the earth?

It is He who sits above the circle of the earth,

And its inhabitants are like grasshoppers.

Isaiah 40:21-22

---

12 Genesis 45:5-8

I sometimes wonder how much I really think I know myself. Do I believe I know myself better than God knows me? Do I think that I can see my true motives more than He can, or do I even know what my own thoughts are? The deeper inward I journey, toward the center of my heart and all its complexities, the more I realize that I hardly know myself at all. As Paul says, I do what I do not want to do and don't do what I want to do.[13] I cannot trust my own intentions, let alone my own desires. Any moral convictions that I believe and which motivate me are rarely more than self-interest. He knit me together in my mother's womb; my frame was not hidden from Him,[14] yet I think I can see clearly. He searches me and knows me, better than I even know myself. But still, I think I am at a vantage point to accuse Him of being unfair with me.

Behind this temptation to become bitter is a lie from the devil that declares that God is unfair. How can God be fair when it seems that He deals with me so differently than with others? I measure God with weights and scales of my own making. Do I think I can judge whether or not God is being fair with me or that, in some cosmic formula, I can determine who has been given a better deal than I have, or vice versa? And by what am I measuring another's life—or my own? Do I know another's thoughts, their maturity, their posture to the Lord? Do I see myself objectively? Even still, do I really believe that the Father of us all, Who has watched the comings and goings of humanity for millennia, cannot determine my steps according to His best for me and for the fabric He is weaving of all human history?

His ways and thoughts are not ours (Isa. 55:8-9). How can I sit in judgment of Him? My story is no one else's story. My sins, my particular combination of weaknesses and strengths, my personality, my culture, and my time in history are all unique to me. So, how can it be that I expect God to do the same things with me as with someone else?

---

13 Romans 7:14-20
14 Psalm 139:13-16

I think of my garden I left behind in Canada. The rosebush grows hungrily and rapidly after it is pruned to remove all dead and diseased branches. It thrives only after it has been grossly trimmed back. Then its blooms can grow. This extreme care will keep it alive and producing year after year. This pruning produces incredible beauty and fruitfulness. Yet if the gardener took the same techniques and applied them to dahlias, a tender annual plant, we would never see a bloom. Could it be that God, our very Creator, knows what we need in each season of our lives to cultivate us to full abundance? Yet we judge, demand, and command that God treat us the same as others. I compare myself with so many and assume what He is or is not doing, even when I haven't the faintest clue. Instead, is it possible for me to sit in the incompleteness of my life and praise Him? Is it possible that He is not finished, that He is still working even when I cannot begin to see what He is doing? Can I accept that He will indeed prune me so that I will produce fruit in the season in which He has called for it to come forth?

I am a parent to four children, and they have never *not* demanded equality and "fairness" from me. We don't have to teach that to our children. If the two-year-old is pulling a sucker from the candy jar, you better believe that she is doing it with an eye to her left and a glance to the right to see what kind of candy her siblings had the fortune to obtain. We don't know what to be content with unless we compare with others. A dear friend told me the other day that every step toward gratitude is a step away from idolatry. There is such truth there. Can I keep my eyes directly on my heavenly Father as He gives me my portion and trust that is the best portion for me?

Lately, I have recognized how much social media feeds into this soiled human tendency. We get very real glimpses into what God is doing in this particular season of others' lives, and we get overwhelmed by the successes we see. Everyone is winning! Everyone is seeing the fruition of their dreams! God is doing better for all of them than for me! However, when we look at their social media, we see the nice picture at the end of another's season of waiting and get discouraged. We don't see all that came before the picture was taken. Perhaps it's time we turn off the constant inundation—the perpetual noise of another's life channel—and focus on our God Who provides for us in every season, not according to "fairness" but according to His Sovereign and perfect plan for us all.

For Further Reflection

1. In what areas do you feel God is not treating you fairly? To whom are you comparing yourself?

2. How could you practice gratitude for your portion? How can you practice contentment?

3. What social media or other influences can you cut back on to decrease your tendency to look around at others?

CHAPTER FIVE

My Fruit from Solid Soil

Apart from Me, you can do nothing.

John 15:5

In our adopted country, much of the culture is inextricably linked to the land and farming. We have spent the better part of a year learning Chichewa, the local language, and we've discovered that agricultural terms are more numerable than words expressing emotions. They have hundreds of verbs and adjectives to describe each part of the growing process—verbs describing the actions of plucking, crushing, grinding, sifting, airing, and the drying of corn. Yet they have few words to describe grief or joy. Agriculture is the blood running through the veins of the population here, and every injury to the crops is an injury to the people. During harvest, every spare bit of dirt is covered in thick stalks of maize. There are few street corners, ditches, or alleyways that are not taken over by this crop. You can talk to anyone— businessmen or women, doctors, pilots, or whomever—and you will find that they, too, continue to work the land. It's not a hobby; it's survival. It's the way of life.

Every part of the maize is used to produce the year's food. They grind the maize into Ufa flour, which they turn into Nsima. This starchy grain is stored year-round and eaten with almost every meal. The process is complicated and particular to this part of Africa.

Every year, the whole population waits with bated breath for rain to fall in December, January, and February. For the rest of the year, the clouds remain closed, leaving us with an impregnated silence from the heavens. Then it is time for the rains to arrive. Everyone is ready for it. The dirt is mulched; the ground is fertilized; and the seeds are readied for the planting and growing season. Row upon row of piled-up dirt ridges stretch as far as the eye can see. When the rains come, they bring storms like I have never experienced. The almost-daily barrage of thunder sounds like horse hooves. The blasting wind and roaring waterfalls that slam against the ground can quickly blow away roofs, snap trees, and flood fields. In one moment, all is well; and in the next, there is nothing but devastation and moaning. The way the earth brings forth life from the dust each season is rarely perfect. There is toil and labor and disparity between how the people want the crops to grow and how they actually grow. This is the curse of the fall.

Temptation 5—Control

So why this agricultural rabbit trail? When I think about who we are in this analogy, I want to believe I am the farmer. Or maybe I am the seed. Perhaps I am the rain. I put myself in this picture as the one doing the work, the one bringing forth life and creativity. I am the bringer, aren't I? Sure, I may play some parts like these. But I think mostly, I am just the soil. I am the dust, the hard dirt, but I am tempted to act as though I am more. I am not the seed, nor the sower, nor the rain and sun. Neither am I the farmer nor the tools. I am simply the dirt.

It's not that I don't have a part to play. But I must recognize the sheer and utter dependency of my role. When I examine the dependent position of the soil, the same that is required of me, I realize how little I can do to produce good work on my own. You see, I cannot bring forth life from the dust without all the other elements. It is tempting to think I can do it alone because there is much I can do. But in this case, what I do either opens me up to the works of God or hardens me to His hand. As soon as I believe myself to be anything but the soil, I frantically try to do it all myself.

I run around like the wind. I work all hours like the farmer. I pour myself all over the place like the rain, and I intensify the heat of my effort like the sun. I try to be all of these things and produce nothing but failure. When my fear leads me, instead of my loving Father, I become my own bully. I tell myself I should do more, be more, work harder, and make things happen where I don't see anything happening.

But does the dirt stir and fret? Do birds?[15] All that needs to happen in our lives can and will be authored by our Father if we let Him do it. But what is our posture toward Him? Prepared, willing, and ready for Him to work through us; or hardened, frantic, and desperately trying to make a way for ourselves?

Therein lies the temptation: to "DIY" (do-it-yourself) this life of mine. If I just do a bit more on my own, then maybe I will end up where I want to be. It is so tempting to do anything *but* sit and wait for it all to come together in this beautiful symphony—to wait for the rain to harmonize with the sun, to break forth the life from the seed, to grow up and produce the harvest. How hard it is to wait upon Him to do all that He will do in His way and timing.

Waiting is by no means inactive. It takes very real effort to care for the soil. In this way we are also like farmers. We must clear the ground of weeds; we must keep it soft and supple; we must give it nutrients and protect the dormant seeds underneath its top layer. It takes effort to fight off the enemy of our souls who might come and try to take the land. Farmers are never inactive. They are diligent in *all* seasons, faithful to the work of maintaining fields during off seasons. They are ready, eyes to the sky, for when the waters come. They are thinking about many things and preparing in many ways. Yet these efforts are not the source of true life and growth.

---

15   Matthew 6:25-26

Scripture tells us that anything we produce of ourselves is a fruitless effort. He is the vine, and we are the branches.[16] We can produce no fruit—lasting fruit—without His Spirit flowing through us. So, what kind of fruit do we want to produce—fruit that leads to death or fruit that leads to life? How do we maintain our life of faith in the waiting and longing? So much of life continues to go onward; we still have work to do. Let us not grow weary in the season that seems like dormancy.

The Lie—It's All about Me

Who has directed the Spirit of the LORD, Or as His counselor has informed Him?

Isaiah 40:13

I'm not an artist, but sometimes, pictures can explain what words cannot. I remember my well-worn, smudged, and torn notebook as a teenager. For a change, I had decided to buy a sketchbook as a journal instead of a notebook. I still recall the image I drew on the first page. The picture I was given in my heart was sobering and revealing. It was a picture of Jesus on the cross, the world's gaze upon His frame. Up on the hill of death, hanging for our sins—the beauty and the disgrace and the salvation of the world all captured in this one figure. Off to the side, on a separate and smaller hill, was little me, bouncing up and down, waving my arms, and shouting to the sky, "Look at meeeeeeee!"

Oh, Lord, have mercy on me, a sinner (John 18:13). "Is that *really* how I make things, God?" Oh, how I want to make everything all about, well, me. I am the star on the stage, right? I am the one whom this is all about, the one in control. I want to tie up every loose end; I want to assume I know what the God of Heaven is up to and perhaps speed things along since He might drop the ball.

I don't often admit it, but I act as though I believe I know better than He of what should fill my life. I become the god of the story and take God off the throne. I simply think that I can do things better than He can. But the reality is, I don't exist for myself but for God's glory. It is His story about the working of His grace for the glory of His fame through me, the sinner. I am the object of His mercy, not the subject. I am the receiver, not the giver.

I endlessly marvel at the works of creation. Whenever my daughter brings me wildflowers she has picked out of African roadside ditches and abandoned drains, she begs me to hold on to this new bouquet. I clutch them in my sweaty hand until they are crumpled, bent, and smashed up, then toss them aside when she's lost interest enough that I can stop carrying them. But sometimes, just sometimes, I stop for a second and examine what is in my hand. The beauty, the uniqueness, the utter intricacy of the creation I hold in my fingers catches my breath. How is it that this entire world is filled with so many wonders? I think of the absurdity of things like bubbles or steam or dark storm clouds taking over blue skies, and I cannot believe that I ever think I can do better. The diversity and complexity of this world, all woven together like a rich tapestry, is extravagant. Nothing is for naught—everything plays its part in its place, and it all forms a unifying song.

Then there is little me, just one person among billions, yet I want to make my own way instead of finding the way God has designed for me to walk. My pride is astounding in light of the evidence against my plea that this whole story should revolve just a little more around me. The path of the butterfly, the roaring of the seas, and the dancing of the wind in the leaves all argue against my case. No, it is not about me at all. I am part of the beauty, not the whole. I would do better to be a limp leaf in the wind of God's plans than a mountain made of the dust of my own pride. This is not my story to tell.

The story of Jonah reminds us that we will be found and found out, despite all our running on our own way and away from God and all the plans we formulate from our own stages. God loves us; He wants to guide our lives to fulfill the beautiful plans He has for us. When we run away from Him, He doesn't seek our downfall but our return. In Jonah's case, God rescued him from his own disobedience through the digestion of a big fish. Jonah realized his disobedience and chose to jump off the boat and, presumably, drown. Yet in an awesome act of grace, God gets Jonah's attention through a miraculous rescue: three days sitting in an organ of a big fish. Ever thought about how those three days for Jonah felt? Sitting in utter darkness, bone-soaking dampness, and regurgitated silence wondering why God saved him? What was He going to choose to do with Jonah after Jonah had been the one to run in the opposite direction from where God was calling him to go?

Ever thought about how lonely that place in the big fish was, how humbling it would have been to realize that being swallowed into darkness was actually his second chance? Jonah, in disorienting isolation and waiting in that belly, was at a turning point. Maybe our places of darkness and waiting are God's grace to us to help reorient us and to show us our smallness and His bigness. After all, it takes only a second for the reality of God's plans to swallow up whatever world of which we are currently the center. Though we feel isolated in the waiting, maybe it's a season to reevaluate. In my life, my waiting reminds me of my place in the larger story, and remembering the superiority of God saves me from my own self-aggrandizement.

For Further Reflection

1. Are there areas in which you are tempted toward prideful thoughts and attitudes? What truths or practices help keep you grounded in humility?

2. What image in creation has spoken to you in this chapter?

3. Meditate on the marvel of creation. What does it demonstrate to you in terms of God's sovereignty, His power, His plan, and who you are in comparison to His greatness?

CHAPTER SIX

I'll Get It Myself

There is an appointed time for everything.
And there is a time for every matter under heaven.

Ecclesiastes 3:1

I am currently wearing a cloak of regret. It is so heavy, so thick, that it is pulling me down to the floor with every step. I hoped for a breakthrough, to see God end my waiting seasons with the sweet relief of His provision; and without that, I look back only to see time wasted on meaningless striving. For fear of wasting my life waiting, I have spent too much time seeking other people's pursuits, callings, and passions. I have been so afraid to be left standing here vulnerable and without "fruit" to prove my worth as a productive Western female that I lost my soul to relentless activity. I have served; I have given of myself and my soul where God never asked me to give because I was so weary of waiting on Him to realize some of my dreams. In my waiting, I gave in to temptation and allowed myself to get distracted with activities, missing His call to pursue His heart for me.

I watch my kids play hide-and-seek, and it is painfully relevant to my own reality. The three-year-old is hiding, aloft in some small, recessed space. She waits for five seconds. She waits until she can no longer handle the silence, the solitude, the thought of being forgotten. Until, in the suspense, she doesn't allow another moment to pass before she bursts out on the scene. She can stand it no longer, and she reveals her whereabouts before the counter has even finished his count.

That is me. I cannot stand being sidelined, being put in a quiet spot, away from the crowd, stuck in a dark corner. When in a space of waiting, I look for a place to be found in—a place to fit, a place to keep busy—as though it is the place in which I belong. I think of an image I have seen on social media: an onion, with one section taken out and replaced by an orange segment. The caption says, "Just because you fit doesn't mean you belong." In the void, in the hope deferred, my soul wants something to hold on to, a place to demonstrate I have worth, value, and a purpose. Maybe it looks a bit like my dream. So, I excuse my forcible entry into that place with vague reasoning: "I can do the work, so I must belong there." If I can't have what I desire, then maybe settling for second-best is better than nothing, right?

I am agitated in the waiting, and while the world looks on, I fear it appears that I am not producing anything valuable with my life. In the absence of production, in the silence of my own dead-ended desires, there is nothing to show for the waiting, in a worldly sense. In an age when we are supposed to be able to summarize all that we are in a screenshot, in a daily photo that explains our existence, it's no wonder we start to itch for a new plan.

Temptation 6—Go Beyond the Boundaries

The reality is that we do have limitations in our lives. Just as the sea has a boundary where it hits the shore, and the sky hits the sea, and the day is overcome by the night, all of God's ordered creation has restraints. We won't be able to do or have all our hearts desire. The truth is that I grieve boundaries. I grieve that I cannot do everything I want to do. I grieve that there are limits to whom I have been created to be, to what I am called to do—limits to thrive within, not to rail against. I have desires that will not be met, perhaps because they are simply not what God has designed or planned for me. I am limited by my own strength; by my experiences and wisdom; by my stage of life, my location, my education—and on and on it goes.

In every season, there are things I receive and things just out of my grasp. The question becomes, how do I remain content within the boundaries God has placed me in, right here and now? If I list all my limits, I am easily discouraged. But I think there is also a place to rejoice. I can take a deep breath and be reminded that I do, indeed, have a place where I belong, and I am not responsible for it all.

Sometimes, we are to overcome barriers and climb over walls. I don't mean to suggest that is never the case. We may be called to persevere on a difficult, God-given path. However, what do we do when we've knocked on every door, when the doors keep slamming in our faces and we are left with a hallway that leads to nowhere? Is it possible to stand within that empty corridor and not give up hope to keep ourselves from busting down a door we don't belong behind?

David understood this idea of boundaries. He longed to build a temple for the Lord.[17] He desired in his heart to build a place for the ark of the covenant to rest, and he even began preparations for its construction. But God told him no. It was not God's plan for David to build the temple. It was his son Solomon's destiny to do that.

It is all too natural for us to want more and more. Explorers, inventors, astronauts, and human rights activists are born out of this desire. There is nothing wrong with these pursuits, but not all of us are meant to walk on the moon, either. This world is not our home, but we each have a place in it. Therein lies the confusion. We can do anything, but we can't do everything. The limits we have remind us that we were created for more than this life can offer. Our longings can either lead us to rebel and bash our heads against the walls of God's firm plan for us, or they can encourage us to hope in the "more" yet to come in the life hereafter.

---

17   1 Chronicles 28:2-64

Now, David could have refused to submit. He could have done everything to stand in Solomon's way. After all, that was what he saw demonstrated in the life of his predecessor. Saul could not come to terms with the fact that God had called David to take over the throne, and he did everything in his power to resist it. But the call of God is irrevocable, and His Sovereign will cannot be overthrown. It would have been futile for David's peace, damaging to the destiny God had placed on Solomon's life, and destructive to the relationship between the people and their new ruler to follow Saul's example. You see, if we take up the space that God is calling others to fill, no one wins.

For too long, I have tried to fit in places in which I do not belong. I have tried to wear others' callings, only to find myself in more despair than if I had stayed in the stillness of my waiting. Not only do we rob others of the joy of serving the Lord in their own callings and abilities, but we also end up finding ourselves lacking the life and vigor experienced when the Spirit equips us to do what He has called us to do.

The Lie—There Is Not Enough (Scarcity)

The thief comes only to steal and kill and destroy;
I came so that they would have life, and have it abundantly.

John 10:10

The incredible thing about God is that He is enough for all of us. He has enough for all of us. His provisions are limitless, incomprehensibly so. But if someone else gets the thing I want, often I am tempted to believe He is holding back from me, that maybe He doesn't have enough for me, as well. I may not say that directly, but I act like it's true. That is how it works in the "real world." I interpret God through my earthly lens.

Ten years ago, when my husband and I moved to West Africa for a short stint, we were almost immediately invited to a wedding. I was excited about wearing local fabrics and experiencing some of the traditions governing such a festive event. I was curious to witness this cultural occasion and had no idea what to expect. When we arrived at the wedding along with hundreds of other people, we found ourselves seated at the head table. I was simultaneously honored and mortified. From my cultural vantage point, we did not deserve to be at the head table. At weddings in Canada, the most intimate family members and friends of the bride and groom occupy the head table. We were foreigners! But it was their custom, in order to honor their guests. We were given meat on plates, cold Cokes, and other delights that most participants only watched us eat. The majority, even the families of the bride and groom, ate from shared pots far from the bride and groom. We didn't know what our proper response should have been, but we humbly stayed at the head table, ate, and participated.

Later, in the quietness of our home, I wept from the spiritual significance of that event. We didn't do a thing to deserve that honor. Nothing. I didn't birth the bride nor the groom; we didn't raise them; we didn't teach nor train them nor bear witness to much of their lives at all. We hadn't done a thing to bless or help, nor did we even know them up until that point. We didn't deserve to be at that table. Yet we were given a place.

So it is with God. I think that though I am invited into a relationship with God, I am in the "standing room only" section. I think He doesn't really see me. I might well be one of the faceless individuals in the crowd, while the real players—the truly called and special ones, the ones without my special brand of brokenness—are invited on stage to sit at the head table. But the truth is, unlike what is possible or not at our weddings, God invites us all to sit at the table with the Bridegroom. All of our stories are interwoven into a greater story, the story of God's mercy and love of which we are all destined to be a part. None of us deserve it, but there is more than enough room and more than enough provision.

From where does this lie of scarcity come—this idea that God simply cannot bless us all due to finite resources and a finite attention span? There may be many factors, but a major aspect is our constant propensity to look at what others have. I can tell you that comparison is an ugly, soul-bludgeoning game in which the enemy loves for us to participate. There are no winners, only losers. Satan loves us to think that everyone else has a better situation than us.

The tendency to compare has always been an issue, but social media only amplifies our propensity toward dissatisfaction. It has killed my joy again and again. If there could be a theme or tag line for social media, it might be, "Everyone else has it better." Gone are the days of living small, in one neighborhood, where we compared only with our friend down the street rather than with millions of neighbors online. That friend is posting pictures from a recent kitchen renovation. That acquaintance has been working out and is really in shape now. That colleague is going on a month-long trip around Europe. That friend is pregnant again. As we scan our feeds daily, they scream out at us to compare and contrast our lives to others'. They beg us to replace our peace with disillusionment and discontentment. I remember one time getting so worked up looking at social media that I exclaimed to my very level-headed husband, "Look at all the stuff everyone is doing! We don't do anything! Everyone else is living life, and we have nothing. NOTHING!" (Okay, I didn't say that exactly, but the words were rising up in me, nonetheless.)

My wise husband sarcastically ran over and excitedly said, "Oh yes, let's be jealous together!"

Oh.

He went on to explain that my perspective was all wrong. "No one is doing everything. Everyone is doing one thing. One. Or a few things. That's it."

He's completely right. I am comparing myself and my life to everyone's lives collectively and ending up feeling discontent with the portion God has given me. Those lies start to creep in, that somehow God is withholding from me. He is going to run out of good things for me; He doesn't have enough!

It's madness. How can even the most affluent people in the world feel like there is not enough? How can we all feel that we ought to fight for what we want before God runs out? That is my unfortunately entitled attitude.

As I wait for unanswered prayers, for the desires of my heart, I stop and wonder at it all. Instead of pointing my finger and demanding why and when and how long, I need to stop and point the finger back at me. Am I praising God and lifting my arms in worship for what He has already done and continues to do for me? God will not run out of goodness or mercy or forgiveness or love. He is overflowing with kindness. When will I accept His provision as the right portion for me?

For Further Reflection

1. Do you ever doubt your place in God's kingdom or compete with others for God's favor? If so, why and in what ways?

2. Do you sometimes feel "there isn't enough room at the table" for you? How does this scare you into not trusting God's timing and plans?

3. What limitations are you are currently experiencing in your own life? Have you taken time to grieve them? What would it take to accept them?

4. Is there a role, dream, or desire you have taken upon yourself that you are starting to realize is not God's dream or desire for you?

5. What might it mean for you to be more content within the boundaries of your current calling?

CHAPTER SEVEN

Calloused to Disappointment

Lead me in Your truth and teach me,

For You are the God of my salvation;

For You I wait all the day.

Remember, LORD, Your compassion and Your faithfulness,

For they have been from of old.

Psalm 25:5-6

When so much of our story is defined by what we feel is "waiting," it is also tempting to become numb to protect ourselves from the pain of the waiting. I often imagine myself in the Israelites' shoes. Here they were, rescued by the power and might of their supernatural God and moving toward His Promised Land, when they found themselves in a desert.[18] It was by no means comfortable, but it was a lot more comfortable than the idea of dispossessing all of the giants they saw in the Promised Land.[19] Maybe they were scared or overwhelmed, but something caused them to despair as they faced the land before them. God had promised they would defeat their enemies. He promised He would be with them, but they were still afraid they would die in the hands of their enemies.

---

18   Exodus 19:1
19   Numbers 13-14; Deuteronomy 1:19-45

Temptation 1—Going Numb

I wonder how I am similar to the Israelites. Have I become so complacent, so convinced that I will be waiting forever, that I do not even look for God to bring about something new? Have I stopped looking for Him to act on my behalf in ways in which I could only dream? I become comfortable in the waiting, put down my desires, and shrug my shoulders. I become apathetic. It's too painful to hope and too painful to believe. *I guess I wasn't meant for anything wonderful. I guess my days are supposed to be drab and lifeless, limp and limited.*

When I think of my own story of meeting my husband, it was exactly in this kind of situation that God introduced him to me. All my life, I had wanted to "be with someone." I always felt insecure, inadequate, and unwanted by the other gender. Still, I desired greatly to be in a relationship with someone. I had written so many letters to my future husband, so many poems and dreams in journals, it was almost embarrassing. But when I was finally realizing that the Lord was enough for me, when I was learning to be content in His love and to trust Him with my romantic needs, along came my husband-to-be. I was so surprised by the idea that God might actually fulfill this longing, that at first, I rejected the idea of starting a relationship at all.

We face the tension: we want to avoid filling our lives with meaningless activity, but giving in to apathy is not the answer either. How do we balance these temptations, focusing on the good activity God has for us and staying content in the waiting? Therein lies the true challenge.

There is a question I should consider in this balancing act: where do I go with the desires I possess? Until God gives me a firm no, do I continue to come to Him and ask? He does not forbid our asking, our wanting and needing.

The Psalms are rich with the words of longing souls, waiting for God to do what appears impossible. God seems to want us to express our longings to Him. Instead, I hide. I convince myself I don't feel the loss, the bursting of hope, bulging against the constraints of seasons, time, and circumstances. Might it be worse to waste away, faith fading into empty days of numbing activities, than to fall apart at His feet? It is more painful to hope, perhaps, but pain leads me to my Comforter; and in Him, I find relief. If I am honest with myself, I would rather be at His feet, covered with tears and raw with emotion, than to waste away chasing empty comforts, which numb my pain for a minute but don't heal me from the inside.

It's so easy to fall into this numbing tactic, especially in the Western world. I shop and cope. I watch TV. I bide my time planning trips and renovating houses, chasing careers and money—whatever I can do to mask the pain I feel inside. I long for more, so much more; but unable to traverse in the dark any longer, I lull myself with distractions. It's too painful to watch for the dawn; it's too painful to expect anything more, so I let my spiritual life waste away. But what if I wasn't meant for the desert?

The Lie—You Can Have Everything in All Seasons

Before the mountains were born

Or You gave birth to the earth and the world,

Even from everlasting to everlasting, You are God.

You turn mortals back into dust.

Psalm 90:2-3

I wished away so many of my early parenting years. I've blamed many things for this, including my chronic insomnia that started postpartum with my first child, my limited experience with small children, my driven personality. But whatever the cause, I really struggled at home.

When asked how I enjoyed being a stay-at-home mom, I would cringe. Not because I didn't love being a mother, but I didn't enjoy being at home all the time. I never imagined staying at home would take such a toll on me, but it did. The endless hours of being needed and wanted. The mundane routines of regular life with small children zapped me of energy. I let it steal my joy.

I wrestled, trying to figure out what to do with myself at home. I was desperate for community, and desperate for meaning. I hated when people told me to "enjoy every second because this season will pass too quickly." I didn't believe them, nor did I appreciate their romanticizing of a season that was completely undoing me. But slowly, ever so slowly, I found new ways of living in that season. I found a community of other young moms to rally with at parks and splash pads. We had endless playdates, apologizing for our messy homes and rambunctious children.

But suddenly, I found myself grappling with the reality of being thrust into a new season. September hit like a tornado, and I started driving to and from school all day long. I never saw my mom friends because we were driving kids to soccer and grocery shopping in between school runs. We were managing social calendars and disciplining know-it-all seven-year-old attitudes. Oh! It turned out that "they" were right.

Seasons fade into new seasons before we know it, and then our only chance to be in the last season is past. We are left complaining that we would have enjoyed the season more if we had known this new season was ahead.

Life has a funny way of keeping us in transition. We never arrive. We are usually moving out of something or into something. Truthfully, we cannot have it all in every season. With each season comes a loss, a gain, and a "not yet."

I look back at my college days filled with endless laughter, spontaneous adventures, and free time and wonder how I could have ever wished it away. But that time, too, was filled with angst. "What am I going to do for work afterward? What am I doing with my life? When will I get married? When will I find the right person?" That time was not free of questions or confusion or waiting. Yet on seemingly endless Tuesdays with small children, I would find myself wishing I could have just enjoyed that time longer. Why didn't I appreciate that time more?

The beauty of this world is that it is filled with rhythms. There are ebbs and flows, comings and goings, hibernating times and reawakening times.

There is much mystery in this for me. Hidden things come bursting forth at the perfect time, after we thought they were gone for good. So it is with our lives. There are seasons. Seasons of waiting and seasons of receiving. Seasons of deepening roots, of ripening fruits, and seasons of cultivating the soil.

Will we choose to remain in this season of waiting, without fear, and trusting that it, too, is part of God's perfect design for our lives? Or will we run away in disillusionment, not knowing how it will nourish and develop our souls? He Who created the rising and falling of chests and seas knows what we need before we need it. We don't know what seasons are ahead for us. He might be building in us the character that we will need to face what's ahead. But we must remain open to His work, not growing distracted and numb.

Flower bulbs fascinate me. They are planted in the fall so that they will bring life in the spring. They go into hardening soil, only to be beaten down by rain, storms, snow, and cold, so that whatever needs to take place in the plant will bring forth a flower in the spring. God is at work, even though we are the ones waiting. He is always at work. Everything God does is significant and for a reason. If we are waiting, it doesn't mean He is surprised and is up in the heavens waiting, too. Do we picture Him wondering what He's going to do with us? He is already doing it. He is at work in all moments, in all the seasons of our lives.

My middle son, different from me in most possible ways, is quite particular. He is particular in ways that I find quite surprising. For example, for a time, while living on the West Coast, this child refused to wear pants. I thought it was a phase when he was two. I thought it was a phase when he turned three. But even when he was five, every day after stripping off his school uniform, he would race up the stairs and put on his favorite sport shorts. Even when it was snowing outside, he would ask, "Do I need to wear pants?"

Part of me wanted to scream, but mostly, I marveled at his refusal to acknowledge seasons. It could be obvious that it was a pants day, and he would still adamantly refuse to see the reality of the world outside his windows. He would be shocked, disturbed, even angry that he must wear pants again. Of course, now this behavior is excusable because we live in the land of eternal sun, but that's a different conversation.

I see myself reflected through my children, though, and this is no exception. When will I align myself to the season I am in? There is nothing I can do about this waiting. I am waiting, yet there is a whole world out there to embrace. With each season comes a new set of questions and a new set of longings. All longings will be fulfilled in one moment, forever, in Heaven—but not until then. Ever still, there are responsibilities which need attending, relationships in which to pour ourselves, weeds to pull, Scriptures to memorize. Life goes on, and I cannot be anywhere other than where I am right now. This is the season I am in, and I can deny it or embrace it. God works with what is, not with what we wish it was. We have little other choice than that. Denying that it's cold outside while wearing shorts will only get you frostbite.

For Further Reflection

1. Have you stopped believing that God can bring about what you truly desire? Do you doubt He wants you to live a fulfilled and abundant life? If so, why?

2. Have those feelings caused you to grow numb in your relationship with God? How does that affect how you seek Him?

3. Is God asking you to give up your desires to His perfect timing, will, and purpose? If not, is it clear how He wants you to continue stepping out in faith toward them?

CHAPTER EIGHT

The Promised Land

Jesus said to them, "I am the bread of life; the one who comes to Me will not be hungry, and the one who believes in Me will never be thirsty."

John 6:35

Here we are, you and I. Waiting. Longing. Desiring. Hoping. Praying and faithfully watching for God to show up, to provide, to call, to do something we have asked. But what if the "thing" we want we finally get? What if that thing we so desire comes? Maybe you finally got matched with that adoptive child. Maybe you got that career boost. Maybe your kid got their chance on an elite team. Or you got to buy the house you've always wanted. Finally, miraculously, supernaturally, "that thing" you have been dreaming of has come. There is celebration. There is hope. There are shining bright faces and excitement.

But what if that fulfillment doesn't come with all that you expected it would? Then what? Realizing a dream may still bring other struggles. Maybe it creates new challenges, pain, sorrow, or questions you didn't expect. I have heard countless stories of such situations. People conceived after waiting to get pregnant, only to find out that their child was not going to survive life, let alone the pregnancy. Friends realized their dream of traveling overseas on missions, only to arrive and be called back home because one of their parents received a terminal diagnosis. The list goes on. Attaining the "promised land" we hoped for won't remove our need to trust God. It won't mean life will be easy however much we hope it will, and it comes with a whole new set of questions!

Temptation 8—Unrealistic Expectations of a Perfect Ending

So, what if God provides in a way that looks different from what we imagined? We think we know what we want. We fix our eyes on the desired outcome—our child getting married, our financial load lightening, a broken relationship being restored—instead of on God. Then when the awaited reality arrives, we are unprepared for the new realities behind it. After all, it was so long in coming that we hadn't thought beyond it. God had plans after that event we never anticipated.

The Israelites were quite certain they wanted to be rescued from the hands of Egypt—broken bodies, broken lives, slavery that never ended. Generation after generation was pressed down and afflicted by unrelenting oppressors. God spoke to Moses and said:

> "I have heard the groaning of the sons of Israel . . . 'I am the LORD, and I will bring you out from under the labors of the Egyptians, and I will rescue you from their bondage. I will also redeem you with an outstretched arm, and with great judgments. Then I will take you as My people, and I will be your God; and you shall know that I am the LORD your God, who brought you out from under the labors of the Egyptians. I will bring you to the land which I swore to give to Abraham, Isaac, and Jacob, and I will give it to you *as* a possession; I am the Lord'" (Exod. 6:5-8).

Hallelujah! God was answering Israel. Israel had been asking, pleading, waiting, and hoping for God to rescue them for hundreds of years. Hear that? Hundreds. They thought they wanted freedom; they knew they wanted freedom. But it's interesting to note how quickly they rejected the kind of freedom God provided. It was a freedom that required continuous faith and trust in God. It was a freedom that required them to leave everything they'd ever known. It required believing in *Who* God is more than trusting in *what* He could provide for them. It required continuous surrender and submission again and again. Israel struggled with this new reality. Countless times as they tried to make sense of where God was taking them, they rejected God Himself.

I can only imagine Israel's confusion as they had to face obstacles, enemies, giants, and the wilderness in order to receive the destiny for which they had so longed—the Promised Land.

What does it mean when our long-held dream does not turn out as we hoped? Were we wrong to desire? What is God doing? I find it interesting the degree to which we have to surrender everything over and over again. I thought I gave up what I wanted. I thought I had laid it all in God's hands while I was waiting. I thought I had let it go. But then He answers the desire of my heart, and I think I can rest here in the space of receiving. I think I can simply have it and that I no longer need to trust God for it.

Friends, we live on this side of Heaven. There is no happily ever after until we arrive there, in His arms, for eternity. Until then, we need to alter our expectations. Struggle is real. Life is broken. The cross is evidence enough that we will face death; we will face suffering, pain, and sorrow on earth. Desires will ebb and flow like the tides, just as the seasons of our lives will fade from one to the next. We will get, and we will lose; and we will do it all over again. But He alone is constant. The fulfillment of one desire often becomes the gateway to new desires.

Unless we recognize that the fullness of all our longing—the realization of all our dreams—can be found only in Him, we will always come up disappointed. We will cry like the Israelites, "We want to go back to Egypt!" *Wait a second, God. This isn't what I was really asking! This isn't what I really wanted! You want me to continue to depend on You? I know You provided this, but can I add a few things?*

So often, I think I've submitted to God, but then I turn a corner and find myself in the thick of self-dependence again. You see, we are wired for self-reliance. We will always lean toward finding our own way—seizing control, taking the reins, and fighting for the driver's seat. We gain traction in one area and find ourselves blindsided in another.

The truth is we don't see it all like God does. He sees us in our entirety—our weaknesses, strengths, hopes, desires, and yes, the weight of those things for which we long. But will we trust Him, continuing to surrender to Him, in the waiting *and* in the receiving?

The Lie—That God Is Only Working for the Outcome, Not in the Process

"You are a God who sees."

Genesis 16:13

Human nature is rarely more exposed than in the emergency room waiting area. Who doesn't understand the unique torture of waiting to see a doctor? It brings out every form of impatience. There's eye-rolling and heavy sighing, demanding pleas and upset stares. You're sick; you hurt yourself; or your symptoms otherwise require immediate attention, and you have to face the inevitable wait at the hospital emergency room. No one likes this. We do our best to bear it. It is especially awful because most of the time you have no idea what is going on or for what you are waiting.

As an ER nurse, I try to inform patients of what exactly is holding things up, but we nurses have little ability to control or predict wait times. Most patients have the misunderstanding that it's like customer service and that the "squeaky wheel gets the grease." Unfortunately, that's not true. Even arriving by ambulance doesn't give you priority.

Every patient is categorized based on an acuity rating, which determines how fast you will be seen. It may be the worst cut you have ever had, but compared to other emergencies, it might be the least urgent. Every second, someone else gets sicker, or a new case walks through the door, the waiting patients are bumped back in line, again. It's maddening—for patients and for nurses. I know patients also get frustrated when they see nurses conversing, sipping their water slowly, or appearing and disappearing for coffee breaks. I sense the evil glances in my direction, even though most of my twelve-hour shift is spent running around frantically.

But actually, there is a lot going on behind the scenes that patients don't understand. They don't see the whole picture. They don't see the nurse checking and re-checking to see if lab results are up on the computer. They aren't aware of the child having an allergic reaction in a different part of the department, demanding the quick actions of many nurses. Waiting patients can't watch the doctor stitching hands back together behind closed curtains. They don't see nurses helping with a resuscitation or delicately delivering bad news to another waiting family.

Patients don't understand all the needs that are simultaneously being met or even all that is being done on their behalf. Most care happens behind the scenes: liaising with specialists, communicating with pharmacists, expediting lab test results, looking up research studies on appropriate treatments, etc. Of course, mistakes do happen in emergency rooms. Paperwork gets missorted or lost; orders fail to get put into the computer; medications are not given when they should be; and people wait longer sometimes because of these human errors. But this is the exception, not the rule.

I mistakenly act as though waiting for God is like waiting for a doctor. I think I've been put to the back of the line, and I am simply being looked over. *Maybe there isn't healing awaiting me. Does He see me behind that closed curtain? Am I forgotten in chair A or stretcher twelve? Does He care about others a little more than me, or do they "get seen" first because He deems them more important?*

Or maybe I think I need to be more demanding. *If I pray a little more, if I try to get His attention, He'll act just that bit faster.* We hate waiting and feel like it's wasted time. But He is working on our behalf, always. We are His number one priority, along with everyone else. He is perfect in all His ways toward each of us, and none are neglected for another. We are all valued in His sight, such that Scripture says He knows the number of hairs on our heads[20] and the number of our days.[21] We all are His top priority. We may be waiting, but that does not mean He is not acting. Much is being done—things beyond our understanding and sight.

I think back on all that had to align for my husband and I to meet. Even that one moment in history was preceded by many other moments. First, I went on a student exchange in eleventh grade and traveled across the country to the capital city. This planted the idea in my mind to go cross-country for university. Next, I was denied entry to my dream internship, but that allowed me more time on my university's campus. Then one afternoon, the Christian club on campus decided to advertise in the park. This led to one moment when I decided to check out the club's table, walked across the campus field, got a free soda, and learned about the club's weekly meetings. A desire planted years before, to sing on a worship team, led me to sign up to join the club's band.

The summer before, my then-future husband had learned guitar to be able to fill the worship leader position. And so, we met—on a worship team, across the country from my hometown, an hour from his hometown, his final year, my first year, our first time being on a worship team. Think of all that was planted, all that was destined, all that was designed for that one moment in history, which has now led to sixteen years of marriage and four children.

Is God not faithful? We think we are waiting just for the outcome we desire. Getting the outcome we wanted is not the only proof that God is working. He is working along the way, to capture our hearts, pursue us, call out our giftings, grow our callings, develop our characters, and pave the way for our destinies. He is not long in keeping His promises. We will see His

---

20 Luke 12:7
21 Psalm 139:16

loving hand in our lives as we wait faithfully on Him. His work is not just the outcome for which we long, but His work is also guiding us on the journey toward it.

Life is filled with these moments that become an entire life-long story. God is at work in a million ways. It's unfathomable to think about all that He ordains in His perfect timing. Why should we fret or fear the waiting as though He is not also working in the middle of it? We are not being passed over; we are not being missed because of lost paperwork. He does not make mistakes like humans do. He does not delay because He's taking an extended coffee break. He is not limited in how many people He can care for, nor does He need to consult with specialists who know more about a particular area than He does. He is perfectly able to meet all our needs in His perfect timing and way.

Praise God we are not in some celestial waiting room for the King's attention! We can be in His throne room, being comforted by His Spirit along the journey as we look for ways He is already working in our lives. He is able. And His Sovereignty will not be held back by our impatience or another's higher acuity.

We can have faith in these truths, but often faith, in this reality, is a lot harder than it seems. What does it look like? What does it feel like?

Have you ever been rock-wall climbing before? If the climbing itself isn't treacherous and terrifying enough, I find it by far the easiest part. You don't have to look down. You don't have to see how far you might fall. You just have to reach up toward the next handhold. Look up and ignore the thoughts of plummeting to the ground below. Simply grab the next hold. And the next.

But then you reach as far as you can go. Your arms are burning; you're tired; and it's time to go down. How do you go down? No problem—just let go of the wall. I remember the first time I did this and recall my unwillingness to remove my tight grasp on the holds. The person who was belaying for me kept saying, "Just let go! Let go of the wall and lean back!"

My response was, "No, thank you. I'll just stay up here, holding on for dear life. I'm quite comfortable doing this from now on."

"No, I've got you! I've got you."

"No, you don't. I've got me. Don't you see I'm holding *myself* up against the wall?"

After a series of arguments on my side, the belayer somehow convinced me that it was in my best interest to let go of the wall. It wasn't a graceful drop, mind you. It looked a lot like a cat clawing up a frozen waterfall. Scratching fingers, slamming limbs, a bit of howling. But then you know what happened? I let go.

I leaned back, and with a gasp of fear mixed with exhilaration, I felt that he did, indeed, have me as I fell. That is what faith feels like. It goes against everything we feel in our flesh. It feels unnatural. It is simultaneously terrifying and exhilarating.

I am enthralled by the story of Joshua lately. I have struggled with a dependence on sleeping medication for over ten years. It's a long story, a long journey, and it's not over yet. I have tried to loosen my dependency. I've tried and gotten so close but then have shrunk back in trepidation. I've cried with the Israelites "the enemy is too great."[22] I've thought I had faith when I was, in fact, clinging to my own power.

But here I am again. Face to the wind, looking at the promised land but suspended between what's behind and what's ahead. I don't see a way through. My natural feeling is to run away from the narrow path. *Go back! Egypt, I want you! Wasn't it so good being a slave? Wasn't it better than this needing to trust Him every, single, day?*

We must trust while in the in-between that God is still holding us up, still working even when we cannot see. This level of faith is impossible without His help. Even faith is a gift! But so many times in life, this belief in God's ability to do what we cannot is what ends up sustaining us in the end.

---

22 Numbers 13:31-32

My God has me. He is saying to let go of my methods and follow Him at every step of the journey to the promised land. Trust. Believe. The even better news is that He doesn't abandon us in the wilderness of our waiting for the promised land. He isn't too busy caring for other people first. He provides for us throughout the journey and is with us ever still.[23]

For Further Reflection

1. Think and meditate on moments in your life that seemed ordained supernaturally by God. Write them down so that in times of waiting, you will remember how faithful God has been to you.

2. Looking at those moments, what do you notice?

3. Meditate on Deuteronomy 32:4: "The Rock! His work is perfect, For all His ways are just; A God of faithfulness and without injustice, Righteous and just is He." What speaks to you from this verse, right now?

4. To what degree do you feel like you have surrendered and submitted your will to His?

5. What are you seeking in "that thing" you desire? What need is underneath it?

---

23 Deuteronomy 2:7

CHAPTER NINE

Idols at the End of the Rainbow

Why are you in despair, my soul?

And why are you restless within me?

Wait for God, for I will again praise Him

For the help of His presence, my God.

Psalm 43:5

As I perpetually seem to roll from one waiting period in my life to another, I realize that I have often skirted around this question of idolatry. I've avoided it, really. It's easy to look at such a word and imagine that there is no way my *good* desires have taken such a hold of me that they have become idols. "Of course, I'm not worshiping that in place of God." But it's time I look at this question and truly examine my heart.

Temptation 9—Putting Our Hope in Getting What We Want

It is so easy to imagine how much better my life would look if God gave me what I wanted. It's so easy to imagine that this thing I am waiting on God for will bring me true contentment and satisfaction. There are many good things we find ourselves looking for—our career to take off, retirement, the right living situation, the right partner, a needed treatment, financial assistance, or another particular need to be met. Yet if we believe we will be happiest or most fulfilled or most valuable to God if we have "that thing" we are waiting for, then our affections have already been sold out and are not placed firmly on God alone.

God's good gifts are never meant to replace Him, the Gift Giver. If I truly worship Him, and Him alone, then I can be content. But am I?

For me, that's the idea at the center of my struggle—that I will not be pleasing to God unless or until I am able to do or have "that thing" I want. But what more do I actually need other than Christ Himself? What am I adding to the Gospel of grace that God has not already given? Can I only be purposeful and serve God most fully if I have children? Can I only be satisfied and please Him if I am healed? Can I only bring glory and honor to Him if I serve Him in that ministry He seems to be keeping from me? Can my desires for these things—or whatever I'm waiting for—be trusted if I am hanging those kinds of expectations on them? Or might it be that God has already given me everything I need to be obedient to Him in this season?

My true feelings and affections are revealed when I lose something or must wait for it. I start to feel panic, loss, fear, confusion, hurt, bitterness, and anger rising in me over unmet desires. These striking emotions reveal the true place this thing holds in my life. If my hopes, well-being, sense of contentment, joy, and satisfaction are shaken because of not having something, then God does not have His rightful place in my heart. Ouch.

What if what you are waiting for never happens? What will that change about how God sees you? What will that change about how you see Him? What will that change about your identity in Him? What do you think that will change about your position as God's child? The truth of the Gospel is that our identities should be rooted in Christ regardless of what we do and what we have, lest we boast in self instead of what Christ has done.[24]

If your answer is like mine, and you are left with a wake of emotions that are anything but godly, you may be waiting for and worshiping an idol.

---

24 Galatians 6:14

Feeling emotion is not sinful, but our emotions are symptoms and indicators of what might lie beneath, like these idols. Idols that, if we are not careful, will not only fail us if we get them but will also change the trajectories of our lives as we wait for them. We may end up running completely off course. God might be withholding them from us in His mercy, giving us a chance to change our hearts—before we lose our hearts.

I find this hard to admit to myself. I think that by pretending something is not an idol, by putting spiritual terminology on it, or by speaking about it as if it's not a big deal, I can fool God. But He knows. Either God is all and is in all, or He isn't. He is a jealous God, a God Who requires that we rest on Him and Him alone for salvation. Not works, not things, not dreams, but Him alone. The Bible calls Him an all-consuming fire.[25] If we have God, we should be satisfied in Him, and Him alone. He is my Anchor, my Stability, my unchanging Foundation. Even when desires and circumstances change around me, He never will. If I am only satisfied in anything other than Him, I will end up disappointed.

I'm not suggesting every waiting period happens because God is trying to tell us "that thing" has become an idol. In the stories of Noah and of Elizabeth and Zacharias, the characters waited upon God, but not because they were unrighteous or idolatrous. It's worth examining, though, isn't it? It's worth considering that everything we desire has the potential to become an idol.

The Lie—There's an End to Our Waiting

My soul waits in *silence for God alone;*
From Him comes *my salvation.*

Psalm 62:1

I remember another time in my married life when my family and I lived in a rural village in western Africa. We were hundreds of kilometers away from the capital city. There was limited access to supplies. We didn't shop;

---

25 Hebrews 12:29

there was nothing to buy. We didn't do anything for entertainment; there was nothing to do. Everything was slower, simpler, and less consumer-based. On the occasional trip back to the capital city for groceries and the like, everything tasted and seemed so incredibly delightful. Imagine going out to a restaurant where food is prepared for you and not from a can! Imagine grocery stores stocked with food! Imagine new books to read! Everything was wonderful after having to wait for it.

The longing, expecting, and hoping heightens the experience of the thing for which we waited. We've structured our modern Western society to avoid waiting as much as possible. We eliminate the joy of anticipation, the satisfaction in receiving something waited for and earned. Gone are the days of "saving up," and with them, the experience of the in-between time. If we want it, we get it. We'll pay for it later.

But where do we find joy and satisfaction if the end of our waiting doesn't come? Or what if the end doesn't satisfy us as we expected? As soon as we get what we want, we often have to let it go all over again in unexpected new ways, to new depths. If we rely on what God gives more than on God Himself, we will still be longing in the end. Because the trusting never ends. We will always and forever need Him more than anything else we think we need.

The problem is, the line of satisfaction keeps moving. We hope and wait and long for something; we get it, and we realize that there are other things we now long for that we didn't before. If we wait to find joy only at the end of the rainbow, we find that we missed all the opportunities for joy in between. Perhaps I think that I need a new career. Maybe I have been waiting for the right chance to pursue it. After waiting and waiting, I finally get my chance. I work hard. I go after it. But after I have it, I find that others are further along than me. Maybe now it's not enough to have that career; now, I want to be the most successful, the most accomplished, the most of something else. Tell me, when will I be content?

The enemy wants to sell us the lie that our contentment, joy, and satisfaction can be found only *there* and cannot be found *right here.* In the anticipation of what God is going to do, in the longing of what is yet to be seen, in the tension of being present in this moment while hoping for another, can we find our joy? The reality is, there will always be something for which we are waiting, and the enemy knows that. If we can't find our joy right here, maybe we never will.

I think of Solomon. He was a man entrusted with wisdom by God. In all his wisdom, he saw the striving of humanity and said, "All was futility and striving after wind" (Eccl. 2:11). Even in pleasure and joy and accomplishment, it is all chasing after the wind. There is never a sense of arrival. Solomon had great wealth and success, and he became the greatest king of his time. Nothing he desired was beyond his reach, and even in the position we might consider "arriving," he still states that it is all vanity and meaningless striving. What does that tell us about what awaits at the "end of the rainbow"?

Yet our longings are real. Our unfulfilled desires are real. Is it possible to be faithful in this moment, to experience hope now, while simultaneously experiencing longing? Perhaps we will never live out from underneath that tension.

Maybe, just maybe, we *can* have both experiences at once. Both are, in fact, part of the story of the cross of Christ. Hope has come; a Savior has come; and His salvation is completed at His death. So, the kingdom is already, but it is also not yet. We are still waiting for Christ's return to make all things right. There is joy and hope but also the lived reality that all is not quite right. I wonder at this contradiction. There is waiting and longing, but also receiving. The now and not yet. Expectant hope, being still and pondering the joy and anticipation of what could be. This is sacred space, a space that cannot be summarized in words or pictures, a space that is unfamiliar and alien to our human nature.

It is possible to find joy in the waiting. I think of a mother expecting a child. The child is already there; the child is with her, but she has not yet beheld the child. There is comfort because she knows she is with child, but the child is not yet *with* her. There is profound anticipation but also the possibility to feel joy while waiting for that anticipated birth. So it is for us. We can wait expectantly for good things from God; we can rejoice in what He has already done for and in us; and we can recognize that the hard times of waiting are not the whole story. He is not finished with us.

For Further Reflection

1. What does contentment look like for you? Emotionally, spiritually, physically, or otherwise?

2. In what ways are you living in the "already but not yet"? Where do you feel the tension in your life?

3. Where might God be asking you to settle into the in-between?

CHAPTER TEN

God Knows Us Best

I have loved you with an everlasting love.

Jeremiah 31:3

In our current backyard in Malawi, there is a hammock. It's beautifully made, vibrant with many colors, and hails from a long-forgotten Costa Rican honeymoon. It spent the better part of its life in a box, while my husband and I moved from rental suite to rental suite, without a yard to place it in. Finally, we became adult enough to dust this honeymoon souvenir off, and it made its way to the great outdoors.

First, it swung between two trees in our yard in Canada. Then it was hauled, with an embarrassingly large number of other storage bins, to this foreign land. One of the first things we did in this new subtropical zone was to hang up the hammock. I guess that means we're staying for a while, though my heart isn't ready to say that is the case.

To be honest, I didn't sit in the hammock right away. Maybe the reality of our presence here and the losses of the life left behind have still been too raw for them to coexist together by my sitting in it. But the other day, I finally sat down, only to notice that the beautiful cloth was covered in little, vibrant-green cones.

At first, I was horrified that something related to insects was infecting my cloth, but then I became a little curious. Upon closer inspection, I could see that little larvae were tucked inside delicate, transparent envelopes of fragile skin. They were little cocoons. Some were hollow, empty reminders of butterflies that had emerged and were living in the air, fluttering about as they were meant to do. Yet most were still inside their temporary abodes, awaiting the big moment when they would burst forth and fly away with newfound wings. I had never before seen a cocoon so close. It was actually quite small and useless-looking, though beautiful in its fragility.

I have been pondering hard, at this stage of my life. Call it introspection, a midlife crisis, or some kind of crossroads, but in this season of waiting, yet again, I am seeing myself differently. I am finally seeing the cocoon I have been living in for what it really is. Self-doubt is wrapped around me like that cocoon, woven with fear and shame. You see, for most of my life, I have doubted my worth in Christ. I have been so busy performing to the choreography of "should" and wondering if I fit in and am living up to the expectations I have for myself that I have not done the inner work that would bring me freedom. And so, I am imprisoned, dying to be released, but I haven't been convinced until now that I need to leave the cocoon. It's not safe for me in there any longer. The cocoon itself is not the truth about who I am. God is calling me out into the wild to grow into the truth He has spoken over me, and I am becoming less trusting of the cocoon of doubt in which I have been wrapped.

Temptation 10—Doubt Your Worth

In all the waiting and longing for the cries of our hearts, it is easy to get trapped in unbelief about who God says we are. Our circumstances come to define us, or we allow them to speak over us. It is so easy to doubt that there is something greater ahead. We convince ourselves that we will be in this cocoon forever, that we are not worthy of life beyond it. We start to doubt that we were made to be butterflies after all. We forget there is a greater destiny calling us. Then we build lies around ourselves that are fragile and hold us back. Maybe we tell ourselves that we are not worthy or chosen enough. We might tell ourselves that we are being punished, or God doesn't love us after all. Our circumstances start defining our worth more than the Word of God does. Perhaps that's the most revealing indication that we have more internal work to do than we thought. Are we willing to do this inner work while we wait, so that when it's time to take flight, we are free and ready to shed the cocoon?

Who gets permission to tell us who we are, anyway? I am realizing that others can't be trusted and my circumstances certainly can't be. I no longer believe I am loving enough or gentle enough with myself to trust my own voice to define my worth, either. Only God's words about me are what matter—do I believe that?

You see, when we experience waiting and see how others are living, we start to believe that maybe we aren't as loved or aren't as special to Him. None of this is true, but it feels true. So, we wrap those beliefs around ourselves and become imprisoned. If God brought the right timing, would we even know that it's time to emerge and live freely in the skies, or would we be found trapped in lies about who we are, unable to even accept His gift?

The Lie—The Belief that God Has Overlooked Me or Made a Mistake

"For My thoughts are not your thoughts,

Nor are your ways My ways," declares the Lord.

"For as the heavens are higher than the earth,

So are My ways higher than your ways

And My thoughts than your thoughts."

Isaiah 55:8-9

I had a question that was burrowing so deep down into my soul that I couldn't shake it. It established roots, spreading its shoots wide, until it burst through the surface and stood tall as a grand oak tree. Bigger and bigger it got, until I couldn't walk around it; I couldn't get out from underneath it. In fact, I set up camp beneath its heavy branches and would not leave its growing shadow. I needed an answer. It was a strange question to articulate, but not so strange if you understood the history behind it: "If God is so powerful, why can't He change the past?"

At the time I was in the middle of nursing school and up to my elbows in textbooks, learning about diabetes and psychosis, practicing injections and sterile procedures. I was also a newlywed, living in a tiny hovel of a basement suite with very little natural lighting. We thought it was a quaint space because we were newlyweds—even though we had to duck to step into the kitchen. And if we rolled a ball from the kitchen to our bedroom, it would go downhill. Each day, I was trekking along public transit lines for hours, trying to make it to classes while my husband worked.

One hobby we enjoyed together was playing soccer. I was a self-reported soccer star. Or, at least, I thought I was because I had played my whole life and considered myself brave enough to play against "the men." Except I was five feet, two inches tall (and still am, actually) and, although competitive and good at egging on others, I wasn't a fitting match for grown men. I'd only ever played with other women. In my attempt to prove I was capable and strong, which as it turns out has been the reason I've done most of everything in my life, I ran around the field like I owned it. Until, that is, I got kicked by a giant midfielder straight in the calf. Just like that, I was on the ground.

I was hobbling for days, and the pain wouldn't go away. Meanwhile in nursing school, mid-lecture, I was learning about leg clots, heart failure, and cardiac arrest. I finally sought help at a clinic, only to discover that I had a clot in my leg. Aren't I the nurse, and "they" are the patients? Shock turned into annoyance as I had to trek to the hospital and endure long ER waits to receive my daily injection of blood thinner.

That began a long journey of discovering a previously unrecognized blood clotting disorder—weeks of self-injections, medication, and appointments with specialists. One year later, still not having shed my desire to prove my worth on the soccer field, I was back at it again. Only this time, trouble came when I stopped the ball in one direction and turned to run in the other. I felt quick as lightning. Unfortunately for my knee joint, my hips turned in a different direction than my knee was facing. I was back to the emergency room, only this time with torn ACL and MCL ligaments in my knee and another blood clot. What came next were months of recovery; learning how to walk; surgery; knee braces; physiotherapy appointments; and crutches. I was left with so many questions about what this blood-clotting problem would lead to in the future. I was afraid.

There we were, new in our marriage, with me freshly certified as a nurse, and all I could think about was our dream of having children. What would this blood-clotting disorder mean? Would I be able to have kids? We were told that likely, even if I could get pregnant, I would have to have injections every day of the pregnancy to thin my blood and prevent clots.

I can't tell you the heaviness of that time. It was real. Palpable. I had so many questions about the future. Why did God allow this? Why couldn't He go back and erase those events so I could start again? Since the incidents themselves determined my diagnosis, I wondered where exactly God was when they happened. The thought of needing to have injections daily to have children seemed impossible to me.

Fast forward to the tree, the oak that I was living under. I had this nagging, unrelenting fear that perhaps all of this had happened without God's awareness. Perhaps it was some cosmic accident, and now He was scrambling to do something with it.

It was a year later when the fullness of this question was finally articulated in my mind. We were on a bumpy road in Middle-of-nowhere, West Africa. After my knee had recovered, one of my longest held dreams came true, allowing my husband and I to serve in a remote village. We were with an American couple in an SUV. Bumping along the dirty, dusty roads.

This inner angst suddenly fell out into the vehicle, tumbling like a stack of Tupperware clattering to the floor. My questions from the previous years, my pain, my confusion about how God could have missed those moments, which seemed to be dictating my future—why couldn't He change them? Why couldn't He go back and erase what had happened to give me a fresh start? Because I'd had clots, if I ever wanted to have babies, it would be after daily painful self-injections, and that was if I got to have children at all. What kind of all-powerful God could not change a moment in the past for us? What kind of God wasn't paying attention enough to prevent what was coming our way?

During that moment in the bumpy SUV, His answer came like a whisper—yet strong enough to not just flutter my hair while I sat under the oak tree, but to topple it over and rip its roots out in one gentle, powerful blow. It was a beautiful truth that won over my heart like a baby's exhale. And it came quietly from the lips of the most unassuming, introverted person in the vehicle. She laid it down like a blanket for me to crawl under, and it stopped the very beat in my chest. As I raged and questioned and threw confused emotions around, she simply said, "Saying He needs to change the past assumes that He made some kind of mistake. But He doesn't make mistakes."

Phew. Like a balloon releasing its air, the untruth came sailing out of me, and I could finally see. God knows and sees all things. Nothing escapes His view. You see, I had started to think that God was not in control, that things in my life happened without His knowing, without His permission. I was assuming He was somehow blindsided by this situation in my life and was scrambling to make a new plan.

But what if He had allowed it? What if it was screened by His love? What if it was still possible for Him to use it for my good?

I saw the true question I needed to answer for myself: am I willing to trust Him when I don't see the "why"? Am I willing to trust when I don't see the big picture? Do I believe He is working for my good, even in the hard things, even in the things that made no human sense to me?

Years later, I would find out that the early diagnosis of my blood clotting disorder would actually be the reason I could have healthy pregnancies. Over eleven hundred injections later, I held my babies in my arms and marveled at every part of them. I would find out that many women struggle for years with miscarriages before they learn that if they just took a daily injection or knew about their undiagnosed blood-clotting disorder, they could have had the child for whom they longed. Those many years later, as the clouds lifted, I could see God's goodness for what it really was—not what I expected or would have asked for, but exactly what I needed. Those injuries, those clots, were His grace to me. I never imagined I would thank Him for them, but because of them, I had four beautiful children and safe pregnancies.

Recently, I was reading Corrie ten Boom's biography, *The Hiding Place*.[26] During World War II, she was imprisoned in a concentration camp, and her sister's determined joy, despite their circumstances, was transformative. She chose to praise God in all things, even when their cramped room was infested with lice and fleas. Corrie asked her sister how she could possibly praise God for such a horrible thing, but later in their story, you see how those very pests allowed the women to remain largely undisturbed by guards. This allowed Corrie and her sister to smuggle in Bibles and take comfort in reading the pages and witnessing to the other imprisoned women. Those pests kept the guards from wanting to come in, leaving them unhindered in their worship and outreach. It is incredible to think of all the miracles we miss because we celebrate only what *we* think are the "good" things when, actually, God is at work in all things.

The God Who counts the hairs on our heads[27] and knew us even as we were being formed in our mothers' wombs[28] does not forget us. He does not

---

26   Corrie ten Boom, *The Hiding Place* (New York City: Bantam Books, 1974).
27   Luke 12:7
28   Jeremiah 1:5

abandon us,[29] and He certainly made no mistakes in creating us[30] but planned us before the foundation of the world. Even when we feel like nothing makes sense in our circumstances now, we can know that His plans for us will not be thwarted. The light will always vanquish the dark. He is for us and with us, and we can be assured He has not forgotten us, for He is El Roi, "the God Who sees."[31]

For Further Reflection

1. What situations in your life, right now, require trust that God is still in control?

2. What do you think God is teaching you in this waiting season?

3. It can seem trite when someone says that "God works all things for good," but how have you experienced this to be true in your life?

---

29   Hebrews 13:5
30   Romans 8:29
31   Genesis 16:13

PART 2

The Way of the Spirit

Humble yourselves in the presence of the Lord, and He will exalt you.

James 4:10

Still in the Dark

Night after night of insomnia creates an alternative reality. In this reality, without the relief from rolling thoughts and heaving anxieties, emotions take over. With even a whisper in my mind that I might not sleep, my body hits the accelerator on fear. Adrenaline kicks in and, having beaten down a pathway through the forest of my mind, races along easily, firing up everything in my body on its way. Having been in this state of hyper-vigilance over and over, I know its pattern quite well. Fears heighten; doubts grow. Before I know it, I am sweating; my heart is pounding; and I am not any closer to sleeping than someone running for their life. It becomes phobic, this fear of not sleeping, and the very possession of it keeps me from the thing I most desperately need. I cannot describe for you the darkness I slip into, the catastrophic confusion, the relentless fear that penetrates when I am facing another night without relief. It catapults me into weakness like nothing I've ever known. You will find me the next day gripping the couch like I might just fall off, tears coursing down my face with the slightest pressure applied to my nerves and barely making full sentences.

In some ways, the experience of insomnia is no different from waiting. Is it possible to fall asleep as your enemy hovers over with a sword to your throat? Is it possible to look ahead at the gaping darkness of dreams unanswered and yet rest and be still? Is it possible not to fall into temptation and believe lies as you are suspended in time and the shadows wane on? I believe it's not possible in our own strength. It is impossible because we are flesh, and the ways of the flesh cannot battle in the ways a war of the spirit demands.

In the minefield of temptations surrounding us here, in this dark night of waiting, we have a choice to make. We can follow the way of our flesh into bitterness and despair, or we can walk in the way of the Spirit. The way of the Spirit requires us to examine ourselves before walking into the dark hand in hand with Christ. Our desires are real, but His Word is more so. Our hopes and dreams feel right, but what God says about us is more right. In light of our desires, we need to examine Scripture to see Who God says He is and to believe His promises to us. He doesn't change even though our desires might. So, let us look together at ourselves and consider the way forward. Despite the temptations and lies in which we could choose to walk, despite the enemy hovering over us and pushing us to find our own way through the dark, is there a better way? We can keep stumbling in the dark, or we can call out for help and allow His touch to lead us despite the dark.

CHAPTER ELEVEN

Examining Our Desires and God's Timing

The heart is more deceitful than all else

And is desperately sick;

Who can understand it?

I, the LORD, search the heart,

I test the mind.

Jeremiah 17:9-10

I'm not sure where this all began. This idea that if I have a desire for something considered good or godly, it must be from God and is likely to be fulfilled in the way I imagine (and on my timetable, no less!). I am wrestling with this topic because the reality is, I've bought into this belief for much of my life.

You know what I'm talking about. You are wrestling with a desire—something you long for so deeply that in quiet moments you find yourself thinking only of that thing. Like an ache, like a hollow space inside you, the pangs are felt so keenly, in an almost visceral way. And you hear an idea sneaking in, mumbled at prayer meetings and in vulnerable spaces. It's meant as a form of comfort, given as a partial truth, when others don't know what to say to you. I've said these words; I've heard these words: "Well, God didn't give you that desire for no reason."

But from where did this idea come, the notion that all desires are given by God for fulfillment? Is it even biblical? It gives us permission to invite our desires to be front and center in our lives. It gives us permission to refuse to submit certain areas of our lives to God. "Well, if He gave me this desire, it will be fulfilled. It's just a matter of time." Or "I don't really have to let this desire go. I can cradle it in my heart and hands and not give it up on the altar."

I would be remiss to talk about waiting upon God without considering whether my waiting is misplaced. What does it even mean to fully submit our desires to Christ's lordship?

Scripture does make statements about our desires: "Delight yourself in the LORD; And He will give you the desires of your heart" (Psalm 37:4). "He will fulfill the desire of those who fear Him" (Psalm 145:19). "Seek first His kingdom and His righteousness, and all these things will be provided to you" (Matt. 6:33).

What we miss in these passages is the object of desire to which the writers refer. Delight in the Lord, the fear of the Lord, and benefits of citizenship in His kingdom will be granted to those who diligently submit to God and follow after His heart. When we follow after God with all our soul, mind, and strength and love our neighbors as ourselves, we gain something in return: true, soul-quenching satisfaction, fulfillment, joy and peace, hope and strength. He Himself is enough to meet all of these needs.

Do I really believe this? This is a painful reality to consider, at first. I feel the acute pain of loss, of hope deferred, of dreams shattered when God asks me to unclench my fist. "But this is a good thing!" my heart screams. "It's not fair!" "This, too?" Maybe God has made it very clear to you that your waiting will end one day. Maybe what you are believing for *will*, indeed, come to pass. I'm not here to suggest that it won't. However, the real question remains: if God were to ask you to let your desires go unfulfilled, could you do it?

In my journey, I have been asked to let certain dreams die, and God has later resurrected many of them. But some have been crucified. Some have been laid down on the altar and remain in the ashes. It is up to God to resurrect the dead. It is up to God to send a lamb in the thicket for the child of promise we are about to slay in an act of obedience.[32] But if we are laying down our dreams while looking over our shoulder for the replacement lamb, have we fully let go of our desires?

I think sometimes the problem is that I trust my desires too much. I trust them more than I trust the Lord. I believe them to be real, to be directive, to be authoritative. But Scripture tells us, "The heart is more deceitful than all else And is desperately sick" (Jer. 17:9). David cries out and tells God to search His heart and test His thoughts.[33] We cannot even know our own thoughts, our own emotions! I am a jewelry box of tangled necklace chains, my motivations and desires intertwined so tightly with my sinful flesh. Who can untangle that mess? Why do I let my desires be compasses for my life?

Crucify or Elevate Desire?

Okay, let's get really personal. I had a very real desire to have children, a desire that was met by four babies in six years. The process of having those children, though, turned out to be much more difficult than I ever imagined. For some reason, it became very important to me to have my babies "naturally." Maybe it's my generation or the culture around me in Western Canada, where health and natural things are elevated, or my general need to prove myself. But whatever the cause, I wanted to be able to cross through this rite of passage.

However, after my first emergency C-section, "natural birth" became maddeningly out of reach—labors lasting days and always ending in C-sections. I did everything within my power to change these endings. I worked with coaches and midwives, did physiotherapy and chiropractic care, but I could not change the outcomes. At the end of all this hoping—at the end of all the trying and fighting for this desire which seemed close enough

---

32 See Genesis 22
33 Psalm 139:23-24

at hand but far beyond what I could control—came doctors cutting and clamping, suturing and stapling.

This journey of mine was very painful. It seems out of place now while I live in Africa, where babies and mothers die for lack of simple interventions. What a privilege, I console myself, that I was able to deliver babies at all. Yet my reality in that time was grief and trauma. My longings were met with closed doors. The truth is, there was always so much out of my own control. Why would God allow me to have this desire if He knew that it would go unfulfilled? The desire to have natural births is not bad—many of our desires aren't—so then, why did I have such a strong desire if it wasn't going to be "good" for me in the end? Yet that desire gripped me as strongly as I grip my daughters' hands when crossing these pedestrian-filled streets.

I don't really know, is the correct answer. I don't know why, after so much effort and prayer, God did not grant me that desire. I have to believe and trust that it was for my good. Would my babies have died if they had exited the "natural way"? Would I have died? Would there have been disability? Health complications? I have no understanding. I do not know the inner workings of my body or the map of my passageways. I do not know what situation was happening behind the scenes in delivery that might have complicated a safe arrival of my healthy children. What catastrophe was held back without me seeing? Or how much of this, too, is the reality of my broken body in a broken world?

I grieve because it's not how it was intended to be, and I have to live within that reality. My body wasn't able to do what others' could, and at every turn, sin and brokenness taints our experiences. I will never know the full reasons for my broken birth stories. But it is in that space of not knowing, like descending off a mountain attached to ropes, that I must lean back with all my weight and know that I am clipped in and bound to an Anchor Who does not move and Whose ways are high above my own. Who

I am has fundamentally changed because of those birthing experiences. How I relate to those in pain, those whose bodies are "betraying" them, has been altered. We grieve and mourn, and we should, because this world is not our home; and often, we don't understand the journeys we are taking while living in it.

I have wrestled long and hard over this one, so hard, in fact, that I'm just now able to talk about it without crumpling and crying. For ten years, I tended to avoid conversations about childbirth because it was simply that painful. But when I start to believe and truly understand that God is for me, not against me, and His knowledge supersedes my own, I begin to see that I don't see at all—at least, not in full. What I think I want, what I think I need, what I think is best for me might not be.

Perhaps in the greatest moments of loss in our lives, we are actually being saved from an even greater loss. Without knowledge, we are left with trusting. We have to trust that God allows these things to happen to bring us to greater dependency on Him, greater joy in Him, greater purpose in life, and greater ability to empathize with others who struggle. That, my friends, is the footing for our souls: that none of this is in vain. None of it is without fruit if we submit our crucified dreams to God.

Maybe we have to consider that as we wait for what we want, God is revealing to us our misplaced affection. As we discussed before, He might be working in the waiting to reveal idolatry.

So, we must examine our desires. Do they grip us, or do we grip them? Do they bind us, or do we bind them? Who is the master of whom? If we possess in our hands a desire or an inclination and hold it openly—if we are willing to lay it down, to submit it to our Father at His leading—it no longer possesses us as an idol might. The question becomes: how do we do that honestly? Christ did, but it was a war that produced sweat and tears. He willingly went to the cross for our behalf, but His humanity was certainly made visible as He wrestled with the reality of the cup of wrath to be poured out on our sin through *His* body.[34] One cannot understand His words, "'Yet not My will, but Yours be done'" (Luke 22:42) without taking into consideration the blood, sweat, and tears that were behind that strained prayer. He did not say that glibly, without feeling, or without the fear that may well have accompanied it. God the Son chose that path, but as a human coming face-to-face with death, He did not want to die on the cross any more than we want our desires to die. He agonized. So should we in order to test our grip on our desires. If God is asking me, can I let it go?

But what about the times we are meant to follow our desires, and we anticipate the outcome to bring abundant life and joy to our stories? When do we know that our desires can, indeed, be trusted? After all, our lives are filled with reoccurring submission, being called where it might be hard to go and doing things that might be difficult to do. We have, however, a loving Father, Who has created us with works to do and callings to fulfill. He has given us desires that others don't have, which He alone has entrusted to us so that we might reflect His creativity and glory in this world. What can be said about the desires that we ought to—and have been granted permission to—listen to and follow?

In recent months, I have been challenged in new ways to listen to the desires and inclinations within my soul in order to know how it is God has gifted me and how He is leading me. I've been learning to give those desires permission to have a say in my steps. I have been encouraged to take even this step of writing down my thoughts around waiting as an act of giving honor to that which God has placed in me.

But how do we know when we ought to open the gates, if you will, for our lifeblood to pour out into the creation of something new, and when we should stop it up and let it congeal? How do we know if we are meant to break down walls or wait for open doors? What posture am I meant to take, in this season, with this desire? After all, these are very different stances: one of sitting on bent knees with hands open in submission and one of donning armor and fighting against all the powers and principalities preventing us from living out to what God is calling us.

The mystery continues; the gray still prevails; the mist covers us all; and we cannot see in full. We cannot judge another's journey any more than we can understand our own. God allows, and He disallows. He opens doors, and He closes them. A broken world gives us limits: some that we cannot fix and others we are meant to push past. And God's timing and ways are beyond our understanding. Therein lies the truth. A person may intuit their desires, but it is God Who determines their steps.[35]

I think that sometimes we simply ought to examine our desires more, in the presence of our God, and keep asking and pursuing until He tells us yes, or no, or not yet. I think that perhaps I don't sit in the desire long enough, nor do I look at it as objectively as I should. Can I lay it all out before God and tell Him the reasons for granting it to me, yet be ready to defend His Sovereignty to myself if He says no? Am I willing to admit to myself that He is able, without my interference, to complete the work He started in me?[36]

God's Timing

While examining our desires and awaiting God's answer, we must also ponder God's timing. Have you ever wondered at the incredible magnitude of timing? How is it that the sun rises and falls in a predictable way? How is it that at just the right time, flocks of birds head south to their winter grounds? How is it that the tide comes in and goes out in a rhythm? How is it that a woman's body knows just when to kick contractions into gear for the birth of a baby? How is it that all the leaves of all the deciduous trees in the Pacific Northwest turn from green to gold to red, then drop in a chorus and

35 Proverbs 16:9
36 Philippians 1:6

synchrony across the landscape? The absolute mastery of timing in creation around us is profound. Timing is important; it is imperative; it is everything.

I remember watching my husband try to mentor an adolescent on our church worship team. The youth was inexperienced, and he'd never played the drums before. Neither had my husband, for that matter, but he was trying to help the young man keep the rhythm of the music, which was the backbone of the song for the rest of the band. Without accurate timing, without accurate rhythm, the whole song would fall apart.

While admiring the beauty and perfection of timing in the created order, I rail against it in my life. I don't like the idea that there is a timing for things. It's even worse when I don't get to be in control of when that timing is. I feel like there is a rhythm I can't quite match, a beat that I can't quite hear; and to dance to that rhythm is clumsy and difficult.

Yet the beauty of timing is incredible—that perfect song matching the crescendo of the story you are watching on screen that touches your heart, the perfect joke in that moment of rising tension that releases anger. Timing is beautiful but only because of the waiting, not in spite of it. When expectancy and hope rise to the point that it might burst like an overfilled balloon if God doesn't intervene, and then He does, His glory is magnified, isn't it? Like a conductor orchestrating a thousand moving parts, we end up with music instead of noise.

Maybe that desire is real; maybe you are ready and waiting well; but maybe everyone or everything else isn't ready. Don't fret. His timing is, indeed, perfect. It doesn't feel like it in the waiting. It feels like forever, like every second takes ten more than it ought. I know the feeling. But if His timing is perfect in everything else in the ordered creation, how can it be any different with us, His prized possessions?

Staying in the Word

I have cared for many patients as a nurse, and I don't remember them all perfectly. However, I recall well one young girl with a rare condition. All the staff knew of her suffering. She had been to all the doctors and all the specialists, and her family members had traveled and researched any possible solutions to her condition. The despair I saw in their complete unraveling was hard to watch. Where do you *not* turn? Whom do you *not* ask? What do you *not* read? What do you *not* do for your child to help them find relief from their suffering? Parents will go to many lengths.

We do not like to face affliction. It can be ostracizing, isolating, and unpalatable. We humans have not always treated those dealing with various conditions very well. It's difficult to see anything that reminds us that we are finite and will all eventually face death. We don't like to be confronted by suffering. I think of the woman in Scripture who bled for twelve years. We meet her close to Christ, not far away. We meet her reaching for the hem of Jesus' garment, pressed in from the crowd, in all probability having to fight for her position beside Him.[37]

Her condition was quite likely a menstrual issue. If so, in that time it would have forced her to be on the outside of Jewish society. She would have been labeled "unclean." She would not have been able to worship in the temple. How did she continue to have faith in God and not grow embittered by His tarrying? How did she continue to follow after Him, when He was so long in coming to heal her? "How long, oh Lord," indeed! How long it seems to take Him to save and to heal! How did she not turn from Him in anger because He took so long to rescue her? Instead, we see her reaching for Him. She touched His cloak. She didn't beg or plead; she just believed and kept reaching for His hem.

Let me pause in this moment and imagine the suffering she had to endure. In a land where water often came from wells, would she have had to daily carry load after load of water to clean herself? The endless work of scrubbing, cleaning, and drying her bloodstained undergarments would have been so tiresome. Did she hide the garments away, afraid to dry them

---

37 Matthew 9:20-22

in the sun? There were no washing machines, no bleach. Was she exhausted and emaciated from the endless iron depletion? Was she cast aside by men, abandoned by family, separated from her community? What kinds of situations did she get into where she had to again cover up her shame? What village doctors or midwives had she seen? Had she moved from community to community, each time having to leave because of newfound rejection? Was she poor from all the people she had paid to cure her with some remedy? I can't imagine such bleeding without endless pain. Was she always doubled over? Did she lie in bed for hours each day? Could she even work? These are abrupt questions in my heart as I live in a landscape of suffering and poverty. They keep me awake at night ruminating on all the possibilities of her reality.

Despite her hiddenness, despite the layers and layers of pain she may have worn like the folded cloth stopping her flow of blood, we find her near Christ. She doesn't hide from Jesus; we don't see her blaming or stoning Him. Instead, she reaches for Him, comes near Him, and grabs at the hem of His robe.

Why His hem? It says in Matthew that she thought, "'If I only touch His cloak, I will get well'" (Matt. 9:21). I think I have always pictured the scene as though it was some grand accident—crowds pressing in, toes being stepped on, clothes being grabbed at, everyone wanting to get close to Christ. I envision the scene. Perhaps a foot snuck in the way; maybe she was tripped and fell smack on her face, and in a last effort to get to the Christ, she grabbed at His garment. But what if there's more to it than that?

I don't think Scripture would mention it unless it was significant. Why does it mention that she touched the hem of the garment? When we take a detour back in Scripture, way back to Numbers 15:37-41, we find that there was a lot of significance to the hem of the robe. We learn that the corners of the Israelites' garments were to have blue, twisted-thread ("tzitzit") on them. They were to be a reminder to the people to obey the laws of God, to not let their hearts wander. As they walked, the weighted swinging of the tassels would jostle against their calves, bouncing along with every step. Step, obey; step, stay my heart; step, keep my eyes on God; step, obey.

Is it possible then that she was grabbing for those twisted corners of Jesus' hem on purpose? I wonder if in her heart, she had been remembering God's Word throughout her suffering, holding tightly to it. And in grabbing His hem, she was communicating, "I have obeyed; I have stayed my heart; I have continued walking in faithfulness, and it is there on Your Word that I cling." I imagine she knew the significance of the robe's hem; she knew the significance of the tzitzit. She knew that God and His Word were her only hope, the only things to which she could cling.

I marvel at her boldness and her determined faith that would bring her out from the shadows of her pain and into a public space. I marvel at her ability to not walk away, despite all the years of affliction. If she knew Scripture that well, it reveals that her desire for healing did not lead her away from her Healer, but toward Him. She committed her heart to Him and His promises. With the years of bloody garments in her recent memory, the weight of all the isolation and exclusion she endured, and the reality of her suffering lived out daily, she found shelter in the Word of her God and ran to Him in her trouble, not away from Him.

Do we examine our desires? Do we let our desires lead us toward the Giver? Do we let our dreams and our pain in waiting on Him lead us *to* Him? Maybe, just maybe, we have those longings in order to remind us of just how empty our cup is and to run to Him to fill it with more of Himself.

For Further Reflection

1. Is the object of your waiting exposing an unmet desire that should find its home in God first? What is God telling you about the desire(s)?

2. How will you react if God says no to that thing you want? What if He says wait?

3. What element of God's perfect timing in creation speaks to you the most? Spend some time observing nature and hearing from God.

4. Do you struggle to believe His perfect timing for yourself? When have you seen God's perfect timing at work in your life?

5. In what ways is your life anchored to God's Word, even in waiting?

6. Where do you see yourself in this story of the bleeding woman?

CHAPTER TWELVE

Examining Our Posture and Position

Behold, You have made my days like hand widths,

And my lifetime as nothing in Your sight . . .

"And now, Lord, for what do I wait? My hope is in You."

Psalm 39:5, 7

It had been over ten years since my husband and I had just been a family of two. We had few opportunities to get away from the kids for a vacation in all those years. The years had been a rollercoaster, a vacillating experience of hardship and hilarity—four kids in almost twice as many years, and the weighing and measuring of time and productivity against their needs and demands. We had battled through endless nights and all the bouncing and carrying and cleaning that comes with little bundles of life. It was time.

We were finally able to get away together on a vacation, to celebrate all the things we used to love to do sans children. We imagined exploring, hiking, new cultures, new spaces, new adventures. It took weeks of planning and negotiating schedules with other family members and friends so that we could manage to get away. Planning meals, stocking the kitchen, giving out important contact information, scheduling who was going to take the kids on what day—I was tired before we even got on the plane. And our adventure away in Peru was truly an adventure. We climbed up into high altitudes and viewed landscapes I had dreamed of seeing since my sixth grade project on Machu Picchu.

As always, when it comes to my husband and me, we found ourselves in precarious situations. On our honeymoon, I thought we were going to die more than a half-dozen times. During this trek up to Machu Picchu, there had been a strike, and the train that normally brought tourists as close as possible to the ruins was shut down. We were planning to walk this portion of the trip, anyway, at the end of a multiple-day hike, so we carried on without issue. Others were not so fortunate. Many who would have normally taken the train were forced on foot. We saw people hauling suitcases, car seats, wheelbarrows, and crates along the train track. With just our backpacks in tow, we were relieved we didn't have the children as it would have been impossible. However, on the way back, after seeing the amazing ruins, the train strike meant that we had to take a detour drive of six hours, instead of the four-hour train ride we had planned.

We carelessly hopped into the car that would take us those six hours, not knowing it would be the scariest ride of our lives. Aside from the emergency births of my children, I have never been more terrified. My stomach was sick with fear, and my face was soaked in tears by the end of the trip. The six hours were spent on a road that carved itself along the edges of a high mountain, beside a deep valley (the reason people usually take the train). It was narrower than a single-lane road but somehow had to allow for trucks and cars to pass each other inch by precarious inch. The road wound around, up and down, as the dark settled in. With every curve, my stomach pitched, and my heart gave way. I do not know how that driver did not drive off the road into the darkened abyss that lay beside it. I couldn't look and could hardly breathe, lest I be the reason we go careening down that valley. I clutched on to my husband until my knuckles turned white, hid my face from the windowpane, and thought of all the ways we were bad parents. *How could we let ourselves be in this position? We're going to die and leave our four children as orphans. All so that we could get away on a vacation? How selfish! How horrible!* I remember the driver grabbing at his phone and my furious prayers for no one to call or distract him. It was horrible.

Yet to my amazement, we made it through the journey physically unscathed. It's a wonder, though, that I don't live in fear like that at every moment. Are we not all perched on the edge of life, waiting to be thrown over the edge at any moment? What is my life that I own any of it? What number of my days can I claim or keep from the Owner of everything? I take a breath, and then another, without recognizing that truly this one could be my last breath—or maybe this one, inhale and exhale. In the end, I am dust, and I will meet my demise as surely as the sun goes down every day in a streak of reds and oranges.

Examining Our Posture

In wrestling with the pain of unmet desires, I have been impressed with the sheer magnitude of the futility of my days. What right do I have to order God to do as I please? Who am I to demand He bring me the desires of my heart and let me live a robust and productive life with all the satisfaction of cold water on parched lips? I have no right to believe I will get all that I want in this life any more than I had a right to survive that frightening drive.

It's a wonder that I ever think I have any control. I wail and fight against the realities of my life, but in the end, I will still be buried in dirt. I see it daily in the sun-beaten land in which we live, in the corridors of hospitals, around every corner, and even in this recent pandemic: we have no real control. We do not choose if we will live or die. The fear of God has been rising up in me, and it feels right and good because my inflated self starts to deflate and I get a better vision of He Who is, indeed, bigger than me.

God's Word reminds me, too, of the fleeting number of my days. We get attached to characters in Scripture—we battle Saul with David; we cry with

David over the loss of his child; we wail with him in the Psalms. Then just like that, David's life is over, and we move on to the next character. After spending chapters and chapters with David, the end of his life is summarized by one sentence: "Then David lay down with his fathers, and he was buried in the city of David" (1 Kings 2:10). Just like that, his life ends. I feel a bit ripped off, like a story with an abrupt ending. *After all these pages I've gripped in this book, after all the highs and lows of this story, it just ends, like that?* Like every episode of our favorite television show, we beg for more, but really, there will be an ending to all things, even me.

Job understood the reality of God's Sovereignty in both his losses and his gains. After his family and possessions were suddenly and harshly taken from him, he was left with the simplicity of these words: "'The Lord gave and the Lord has taken away. Blessed be the name of the Lord'" (Job 1:21). He had a choice of what his posture was going to be. In light of God's Sovereignty, what choice did Job have but to "repent, *sitting* on dust and ashes" (Job 42:6). Our hearts can worship in a fearful respect of God, or they can refuse to bow down. Either way, our lives are not our own. Job's posture remained the same as God restored to him all, and more, of what he had lost. He recognized that none of it was his to cling to or claim as his own.

What will my posture be no matter what God gives me or removes from me? Can I—*will* I—choose to have a posture that is unmoved from its firm trust in the Sovereignty and complete authority of God? Will my posture be one of acceptance or refusal? Possession or submission? I am holding on to mist if I am holding on to my life. Will I trust God's ways, or will I refuse them? His ways will remain the same no matter what I choose, but the outcome of my relationship with Him might be very different. To better understand this relationship, we must also look at our position in relation to Him and His mighty love.

Examining Our Position

Just as a father has compassion on his children,

So the LORD has compassion on those who fear Him.

For He Himself knows our form;

He is mindful that we are nothing but dust.

Psalm 103:13-14

I don't think I could ever bungee jump. Nothing about the idea of standing on a precipice, or leaning forward into the pull of gravity, or diving into the abyss below seems in any way inviting. I have the same apprehension with deep sea diving or space exploration (although I hardly imagine these latter situations will ever be presented to me). The idea of diving out into darkness and emptiness or staring into an endless depth of colorless blue and black is unhinging. Even though no one does these things without some tie or anchor, the slightest feeling of being untethered or unattached creates fear and panic in me.

Yet it is by this fear that I have often lived my life. I feel like I am perpetually experiencing the bouncing of bungee jumping, the drifting off into outer space, or the falling deep down into the dark ocean, while forgetting about the tethering elastic line anchoring me to the surface. God's love is that line. Life is more difficult than I imagined it might be, and I see it all around me.

We are jerked around and bashed about, up and down, but our faith doesn't have to be like that. Our position in Christ isn't meant to be like that. Our connection to Him is not earned or jockeyed for, nor does it depend on us. Christ alone is the Line connecting us to our Father. He will not fail. When I repeat that to myself, it makes me weep. He will not fail. Do I realize it does not depend on me, that He will fight for me and I need only be still?

Ultimately, everything comes back to love, doesn't it? Right now, in my mid-thirties, I find myself having a crisis of midlife proportions, wondering and wandering and despairing of hope that God has plans for me, when at the root of it all is simply just love. Do I trust that God is my loving Father, that everything toward me is screened through His love for me? Do I trust my position as receiver of endless love? In all moments of my life, when everything around me is bouncing and spinning and rolling around, do I remember and stay my heart on the reality of God's love for me, anchoring me? Or have I forgotten that the line is even there as I see only the darkness encompassing me?

His love is as the ocean, its depths unsearchable, its weight unimaginable. I am bobbing on the surface of this great ocean of love, fearful that it cannot uphold me, as though it were only a small raft. But oh, the vastness of His love buoying me up!

You see, He is unchanging. His posture toward us is unchanging, but I sometimes interpret God's character through the story of my life. I imagine Who God is based on what He allows to happen to me or keeps from me. I am looking at the surface of the water to explain the depths of the ocean beneath. But there are realities down below that the surface of the ocean does not explain. The surface does not define the ocean; the ocean defines the surface.

Even if I never get that desire, even if my whole life is spent waiting, even if I don't understand or fail again and again, I am His child. Do I doubt that the tethering line is there and therefore hold back from venturing into the deep for fear that I will not be held? The line will not snap; the cord will not fail; I will not be let go because Christ is faithful. Do I doubt His love from the little I know of it, when its vastness is beyond imagination?

Whatever it is that you are waiting for, do you allow "that thing" to define your position to God, your attachment to Him?

For Further Reflection

1. What is your posture toward God in the midst of your waiting on Him?

2. What do you believe God thinks about you? Why?

3. What do feel is God's position toward you? Where is He in relationship to you? Why?

CHAPTER THIRTEEN

Examining Our Minds and Emotions

And do not be conformed to this world, but be transformed by the renewing of your mind, so that you may prove what the will of God is, that which is good and acceptable and perfect.

Romans 12:2

I have stopped trusting my thoughts as the definitive voice on my circumstances. Okay, I haven't really, but I am on a journey toward this goal. I know less than ever. I think of the arguments I have with my now twelve-year-old—you know, the one who seems to have the *whole world* figured out? No matter the subject, he seems to have an opinion about it, whether it be colonization and other historical facts, electrical energy, or current world politics. As a child, if you remember, the world fits easily within legalistic ideals, doesn't it? There is no imagination for perspectives beyond our own, no recognition that there is a world we have not yet seen or experienced. This is a natural tendency and a normal stage of development—this categorizing, classifying, and organizing of the world so that the whole of it doesn't scare us to death.

But as time goes on, naivete turns to wisdom as we start to realize that more and more situations and people challenge the views we possess.

Examining Our Thoughts

I'm only in my thirties, and I can finally start to admit that I simply don't know what is best for me. I can't say I understand my emotions or what makes me do what I do. I thought I did but not anymore. I can't say that my desires are safe, or true, or divine. I am falling hard onto the ground of my humanity and recognizing my illegitimacy as the author of my own life and story. So many of my thoughts—thoughts I believed were true—are not based on God's Word. Lies that I took hold of have, in turn, taken hold of me, and I cannot see clearly anymore.

In the seasons of waiting, we need to truly examine our thoughts. I laugh with others that if I were left on an island with just myself and my thoughts, I would have enough of a spiritual battle without other sinners even around. My thoughts are a battlefield. What thoughts guide my life? What conversations are behind my desires? What do they say about me? What desires are truly God-given; and which ones are shaped by culture, social media, perceptions of others, or our own expectations of ourselves? What do I think will happen if I receive that desire or another for which I am waiting? What do I believe about God if those desires happen or don't happen? Are my beliefs about God based on Who He says He is or Who I think He is, as interpreted from what He has done in my life?

This is not easy work. It is work that takes place in silence and solitude, in contemplation and soul-searching, in the downward and deep direction inward. We rush past this work because it's difficult and arduous. This kind of work is what we are called to do, but it requires constantly swimming upstream. If I am not actively working against the momentum of my flesh in the raging river of my culture and time, then I will be swept away by the lies, and I will drown in them. Most of the time we are moved about by our thoughts without giving a moment to discern what thoughts we are thinking!

Replacing lies in my mind with the truth of God's Word can be painful because His Word might slice as a sword separating even my soul and spirit.[38] It cuts deep. It can cut through the lies of who I think and feel that

---

38 Hebrews 4:12

I am and expose how different those are from Who He says I am. His Word illuminates that which we cannot see in the darkness of our own minds. God has mercy on us; we are as dust and ashes, and we cannot see as He sees. Maybe the truth is that the desires we think we want have everything to do with our expectations of ourselves or others' expectations of us more than with God's plans for us. Maybe the truth is that I don't like His plans for me and the limitations in my life, and I simply cannot accept that they are smaller than what I arrogantly want for myself. Maybe the truth is that our desires are misplaced because of envy or competition. Perhaps our desires are formed from what we expect we *should* do, rather than the freedom of being who we really were created to be.

How do we start to replace the lies within us with the truth about us? The Bible talks about taking every thought captive, submitting even our thoughts to His truth,[39] and about renewing our minds rather than conforming to the patterns of this world.[40] We need to start the way the farmer does—by clearing the land. Remove all the debris, all that prevents His truth from sinking deep within us and taking root. What do I know to be true about who I am from God's Word? How can I walk into the mystery of what is to come, whether it is what I hope for or not, while never losing my grip on that which is unshakable?

Let us examine our minds, our thoughts, and our self-conversations. There is a lot of noise back there and many voices. Like my ten-year-old following me around with incessant chatter, we are rarely left alone in the presence of God without our thoughts leading the conversation. Let us allow God's Word to lead; let us allow our fears to be silenced; and we might find that the truth that remains is strong enough to hold us up while we wait for the rest to be revealed.

---

39   2 Corinthians 10:5
40   Romans 12:2

Examining Our Emotions

"Let your tears stream down like a river day and night;

Give yourself no relief,

Let your eyes have no rest.

Arise, whimper in the night

At the beginning of the night watches;

Pour out your heart like water

Before the presence of the Lord.

Lamentations 2:18-19

We have to wrestle with our thoughts, but we do not do that in the absence of many strong emotions. I had to wrestle with God, with trusting Him amid my spinning circumstances, wayward thoughts, and doubting emotions when my father announced to me that he was getting remarried. My previous interactions with him during this tumultuous time in my family life were punctuated by high-pitched, angry snarls, emotional tsunamis that would crash down and engulf me and those around me. I was a teenager; I was in terrible pain; my family had crumbled around me; and I was adamantly refusing to allow peace to prevail. My weapons against all the chaos swirling around me were my careless, emotionally saturated words thrown about without remorse. So, in that moment, after my dad's announcement, it was only by a miracle of the Holy Spirit that I had the wherewithal to excuse myself from the room. I didn't trust myself to respond in a way that would be at all helpful. I set out for a walk, and my anger subsided and dissolved into another rush of tears.

As I walked and talked with God, it was a poignant moment for my soul. Anger turned to grief, and my grief found solace in the arms of Someone else who was grieving—God—not grief about the remarriage, but about the loss of my parents' marriage. Together, we grieved what was lost, what had been shattered in my home—not because of people, but because of the world in which we live. We grieved that this life wasn't as He intended it all to be. We grieved that this side of Heaven was a messy business and not the perfection He created.

Grief was my servant that day, guiding me softly into the arms of a loving Father Who had made Himself vulnerable enough to feel deeply, with me, the losses the sinful world had caused me. Grief felt like a sigh in that moment, a wonderful and wondrous sigh. A sigh that was both releasing and gripping. I had not allowed myself room for grief before, only anger, but grief will make its way in whether we make room for it or not. In that moment, though, I felt deeply comforted in knowing God grieves, too.

When we wait, we experience many difficult emotions that we sometimes ignore or sometimes allow to shape too much of our experience. But we need to listen to and examine our emotions. They will give us evidence for what is going on deeper. We experience deep pain, and there is grief that needs to be expressed. We need to study our emotions to understand the thoughts and fear beneath them. We cannot ignore them; we need to make room for them.

Have you mourned that life is not as you hoped? Have you made room for your emotions to lead you into the arms of your Father instead of running away and accusing Him of all that you have lost? We can lament safely in the arms of our Father. We can lament without fear. The book of James tells us to consider it joy to face trials of many kinds because they will produce in us characteristics for which we long.[41] Yet considering the joy cannot be mistaken for running toward trials. This world is full of pain, and we are not meant to embrace it as though we welcome it. We were not created for pain. We were not created for loss. We were created for love and for eternity. It is right that we grieve. It is right that we allow room for grief and know that God is in it with us.

41 James 1:2-5

I love the story of Lazarus in Scripture. In her grief over Lazarus' death, Mary ran out to greet her tarrying Lord and said to Him, "'LORD, if You had been here, my brother would not have died'" (John 11:32). Isn't that the cry of our hearts? And "Jesus wept" (John 11:35). He wept because He was grieving His friend. It was sad. It was horrible. It was sickness, death, and everything wrong in the world. Jesus wept for Lazarus. Now, He weeps with us.

But weeping and grief can give way to resurrection and life. Blessed are those who weep now because they will be comforted[42]—in this life and into the next. God is not absent from our times of waiting; He is not far off, and we are not abandoned. He was there in the four hundred years that the Israelites longed to be free of slavery. He was there while they waited for a Savior. He is here while we wait for His return. He is here, and He knows that we are like children and need His presence to manage all the emotions that surround us in the waiting. He is Emmanuel, "God with us."

I am becoming acquainted with a group of people who know grief and waiting like a mother knows her child's face. A group of refugees, living in a difficult camp, are waiting for freedom. They do not have a permanent home. They have lost innocence and family. They have escaped with only their lives from war-torn countries, and they are sojourners in this land. They have birthed children in this camp; they have lost husbands in this camp, and they are heavy with grief and loss. They mourn against the injustices in the camp—the hunger, the lack of hope and a future.

They are mothers like me, who have desires for their lives. They want education for their children. They want food for their children's bellies. They want what sometimes seems impossible to have. Yet God is near them. God is birthing in them a hope beyond their circumstances. Though many have been in this place for ten years or more, He is awakening in them a belief and a trust that He is not finished with them. And this hope can be born in you, too, in all your dead places that seem forever lost. Even when it might look like your waiting has the final word on your life, it doesn't have to.

Sometimes, it takes truly grieving what could have been in order to embrace what actually is. Can we be present to our current circumstances if we haven't said goodbye to what could have been instead? I find myself too long encamped at the graveside of my desires, bemoaning what could have been rather than embracing what remains. As time passes, we watch dreams slip away or realities take hold that we would never have chosen or imagined for ourselves. We will miss out on what God has for us right here if we do not let go of what isn't here. But we cannot let go until we say a proper goodbye.

I struggle sometimes with the seeming inefficiency of God. But then, sometimes what looks like inefficiency is actually grace. Let us allow ourselves to feel the losses and the pain of waiting, but also let that pain be our servant guiding us to where we can find our only true comfort.

Lamenting—The Art of Grieving

"My cries pour out like water.

For what I fear comes upon me,

And what I dread encounters me.

I am not at ease, nor am I quiet,

And I am not at rest, but turmoil comes."

Job 3:24-26

Lately, I have been learning how to lament. There is a beauty in the rawness and unrestrained expression in the Psalms and many other places in Scripture. David often unleashed all his pain before God in ways that many of us would think were blasphemous or irreligious. How could he possibly get away with talking to God like that? David talked about cruel things he wanted his enemies to experience, deep and dark thoughts he had about himself and God, and depressive phrases that bordered on suicidal thoughts. Yet we see a healing that takes place within him in the process of expressing his true feelings and fears. Lamenting is wholly necessary while we live on this side of Heaven. Without true expression of our grief as we wait, as we long, as we hurt for the things we desire, we can almost pretend that it's not as painful as it really is. But that's not the truth, is it?

The thing about waiting is that it allows us to stay in our pain a while if we let it. There is time to dwell on it, to peel back the layers of pretense and examine what is at the heart of our true desires. As we sit with our desires and the pain of seeing them unfulfilled and bring it all in one big mess before God, there is healing and revealing that takes place. There are many things we need to deal with, after all. If it's not our envy, then it's our idolatry. If it's not our fear, then it's our doubt about our worth. As we take time to lay out what we want before the Lord, we start to notice we have a lot of internal work to do. Waiting gives us the opportunity to pour it all out before God, again, and be honest about it. The tragedy is that few of us take the time to lament as we ought. When we are willing to go to the depths of our fears and doubts to the bottom of our pain and loss, we find that God's love and comfort turn out to be deep enough to meet us there.

For Further Reflection

1. What thoughts do you need to consider in light of Scripture?
2. What are you actually thinking about this waiting period? What are you learning? What is it revealing about your character?
3. Read David's lament in Psalm 130. What phrases can you relate to the most?
4. Take time to write out a lament to God for this season of waiting. Pour out your heart like David.

PART 3

The Fruit of Waiting Well

The LORD supports all who fall,

And raises up all who are bowed down.

The eyes of all look to You,

And You give them their food in due time.

You open Your hand

And satisfy the desire of every living thing.

Psalm 145:14-16

Growing While We're Waiting

We know waiting is difficult, and it brings with it many temptations. We are tempted in so many ways to abandon course, to distrust God, to go our own way, and more. So, what do we have to gain if we settle into it? What can we hope for if we trust the timing and the Giver with the ultimate outcome? Once we have examined ourselves in light of the reality of our waiting season, what benefit can we hope for as we keep our eyes on Jesus?

Let us consider what is at stake for us and our communities if we embrace our seasons of waiting and learn all that we can learn in them. Let us consider the measure of growth we will experience if we walk faithfully forward, expecting God to do great things in and through us, even in seasons of waiting.

CHAPTER FOURTEEN

What Waiting Does for Our Relationships

Blessed be the God and Father of our Lord Jesus Christ, the Father of mercies
and God of all comfort, who comforts us in all our affliction so that we will be
able to comfort those who are in any affliction with the comfort with which
we ourselves are comforted by God.

2 Corinthians 1:3-4

I was a few months postpartum with my firstborn son. I was knee-deep in adjusting to life with a newborn, which was much different than I expected. I was like any new mom—worn out, wrung out, loving my son but learning how to be a mother like a baby bird learns to fly (by falling and flailing in the air without a clue how to flap my wings). One night, I couldn't seem to fall asleep. I remember thinking that maybe it was the iced tea I had drunk. I was even more exhausted the next day having had very few hours of sleep, only to roll into bed the next night with a worsening of my symptoms.

So began a trial in my life that lasted longer than I ever imagined it might. Night after night of insomnia spiraled me downward into emotional exhaustion and depression. I would go days without sleeping at all. I sought out solutions, medical help, and whatever I could to try to get on top of the nightly panic of not sleeping. I was a wreck. I was barely coping. I finally found out that I had a thyroid condition leading to a whole myriad of symptoms that were keeping me up at night, but there was nothing to do but "wait it out."

What started as a few months has turned into a ten-year ordeal of insomnia, sleeping pill addiction, anxiety around sleep, and so many tears. Trying to describe the relentless difficulty of insomnia is much like attempting to describe any battle one faces. Until you are in it, you have no idea the toll it takes. Until it had me in its grips, I never believed it could be so devastating. I never considered that I could be pitched into a world of darkness I hardly knew existed.

I remember one of the first turnaround moments for me. My symptoms weren't gone; nothing had changed in my circumstances. (It was actually five years before I would see even mild relief.) But everything about my perspective changed. I took all my despair and placed it right at the feet of Jesus. I cried out to Him. I came to Him, as James says in the first chapter of his book, and begged for wisdom. How could I possibly endure this trial? I couldn't. All I could do was lie on the couch and wail, cry, and give up. And God's Word became my lifeline.

I clung to it with the very tips of my fingers, like I was hanging from a precipice and the ledge of truth was all I could hold on to. His Word taught me so much: He never promised it would be easy. He promised to stay with me. He is enough. He loves me and has good plans.[43] He was going to use this in my life and character for my good and His glory. The truth rolled over me like wave after wave. I won't say that I never struggled after that point or that I didn't have horrifying weeks and months of emotional turmoil and anxiety—or even that my circumstances improved. But God brought about in me a power to endure my trial that I could never have worked up myself—a power made perfect in weakness (2 Cor. 12:9).

God is the only Source of strength in the midst of our trial of waiting. He is the only One Who knows just what we will need, when we need it, to endure with our faith intact. But the real question is: do we go to Him for that strength, or do we run everywhere else? Do we trust Him alone to be our Shelter, our Anchor in the storms?

I can tell you that I did a lot of crying, weeping, whining, fit-throwing, and help-seeking at the feet of everyone else but God in those first months. I was not eager and ready to accept the trial I was enduring. I fought it tooth and nail. I did everything I could to control the situation, to gain sympathy, to escape, to *fix* it. I was shocked and dismayed. How could this be happening to me? How could I carry on for the rest of my life living with such horrible insomnia?

Empathy in Our Relating

This trial changed me. I do not want to be the person I was before I was plunged into the dark. Who was I before this trial? I was a person who thought I knew empathy. I thought I knew what it was to suffer. I thought I could never be *that* dependent, *that* needy, *that* desperate. Even though our sufferings in waiting might be unique, the results are similar. We are rubbed raw, we are exposed to the core, and we find what truly lies underneath. What remains underneath all our posturing, pretending, and providing for ourselves?

It turns out, under the skin I was living in was a person who was not merciful or kind to those in suffering. In the past, I had been like Job's friends, hurling pity like stones at those who suffered. I was good at passing out "encouragements," like bubbles that blow in the wind and pop under pressure. I did not know empathy. I did not know that those who are suffering already bear a cloak of heaviness and don't need trite statements to push them further into the muck. I did not know that those who suffer need someone to climb into the pit, wail at the heavens, and hold up their questions to God *with* them. I did not know that a true friend sits in grief, counts the losses, and doesn't suggest solutions to the one whose life is in pieces on the floor.

Suffering teaches and equips us to relate to others in their suffering. Waiting teaches us how to have grace for all the other wait-ers around us. We are all in this painful world together. When waiting and longing touch our own stories, we never look at another's story in the same way. That's how we know that God is with us in our suffering. He, too, has suffered, and it cost Him dearly. He knows how to empathize because He has known pain, sadness, waiting, and longing Himself.

If we are not willing to be taught by the waiting teacher, we starve our communities of our true encouragement. What can we offer another wait-er other than our pithy attempts at encouragement? If we have always received all that we wanted, what do we have to say to everyone who hasn't? God equips us to minister, sometimes through our own pain.

The pain of waiting is a reality for most of us. How much we need one another to be honest about the difficulty of this journey we are on! Behind the social media facade in which we are all happily living our best lives, we are a bunch of hurting people wishing and wanting for more. Can we be honest about this? Can we be honest that we are not okay? As we learn to sit in our longings, to bring them to our loving Father, and to be taught by these waiting periods, we grow in empathy and compassion for others in their trials of waiting.

Waiting is a great teacher of empathy, if we are willing to sit and learn. As we wait on God, as we have to be comforted by Him amid our sorrow and loss and longing, we learn to be comforters of others.

A Community of Waiters

Weep with those who weep.

Romans 12:15

While working as a nurse, I've been witness to many significant losses and sorrows. I have seen all kinds of suffering. I have watched people take their last breaths. I have watched people so crippled by pain that addiction is the only reprieve from it. I have seen and heard and sat beside experiences that I can barely watch, let alone care to experience myself.

I have always imagined I was quite empathetic. I feel things deeply and am moved by suffering in a way that nothing else moves me. I have wrestled with what it means to offer a gentle touch, when to be quiet and just be present, and when to grip a hand a little tighter. I have washed the feet of the broken and wiped tears and mess of the lonely and dying. Yet I never really understood what physical suffering felt like. I was the nurse, not the patient. I was the one who had the privilege of getting up from beside the bed and walking away at the end of my shift.

That is, until I started walking these last ten years of anxiety-ridden insomnia. There is no struggle in my life that has laid me lower, or rubbed me more raw, or crippled my strength more than this one. As I write this, I am in the thick of it still. Like waves of the sea rolling over me, every night is a battle to make it through with my hope intact. I have experienced what it means to have a chronic issue that does not seem to let up. The dark and endless nights, the deep waters that suffocate, the endlessness of physical attack won't relent.

Who was I before this? I was a spectator. I knew about suffering, but I didn't *know* suffering. I hadn't met suffering face to face before, in the mirror staring back at me. At least, not in my own flesh. Everything is different now. I have walked hand in hand with despair. I have worn the garments of heaviness. I have been mocked and kicked down by the bully of comparison. I have screamed at the walls and lain depressed on the couch. I have been wrung out and beat down. I *get* it. Of course, I don't get it *all*. But I've lived in the shadow side of life for a while, long enough to see the faces of those walking beside me with a new perspective.

How I interact with people is different. I don't offer arms-reach platitudes anymore, for one. No longer in the stands, I am right on the field. No longer do I offer pitying looks or quick suggestions like, "Have you tried sleepy tea?" I don't tell people that I "totally get what you're going through because there was this one time I couldn't sleep, and it was so hard." I don't try to understand or relate to others' experiences fully. Instead, I lie on the floor with others more. I sit in the muck and stare at the heavens more. I lament louder. I yell at the walls with them. I grieve harder for them in their trials. I wait with them. I don't wish they'd change the subject when they call me about their mental illness for the fiftieth time. I don't judge and condemn when someone is addicted to alcohol after their daughter died.

We are in this broken, messy world together, and it's so thick with difficulties and trials. I'm tired of offering a veneer of togetherness and a pretension of perfection. Life is ragged and raw and hard. We need people to slog through it with us. I'm tired of Pinterest-ifying my life. There is no reason to pretend we are not broken ourselves because we need each other so desperately.

As I began this journey with insomnia, like many who face trials, I started through the typical stages of grief I read about in nursing school. I was angry and in denial about what was happening to me. I quickly sought a solution, a way out from underneath it.

I understand personal bodily suffering way differently than I ever have. I understand better what it means for the hospital patients I care for that have been enduring chronic pain for years, what it means for that mother with multiple sclerosis, what it means for that man with arthritis. I see how it affects any of us when our bodies break down and when we wake up (for some people) the next morning with our whole life looking different.

I think anytime we go through a trial or suffering, even a waiting period, we all start out asking the same questions. In frantic pleas, we demand from God, "Why me? Why this? Why now?" We flail about in anger and disbelief, shock and fear. How could this happen to me? During that first year of infertility, the first year of that diagnosis, the aftermath of infidelity, or the throes of job loss, it all starts out the same. We rail against it. My trial of insomnia wasn't something that started gradually over the course of my life. One day, I was sleeping normally, and the next I wasn't. Just like that.

But over time, as we fall down prostrate, face down on the ground at the end of our fight, when we are humbled and laid low to the ground, we discover that we really do need God after all. When things are going well, we think we are in control of our lives. But when it all falls apart, we see ourselves as we truly are—in complete need of Him, in need of others, just in need.

It's then that our questions start to change. They shift from "Why me?" to "Who else?" If we weather through our anger and allow the trial to do its work, our eyes move off ourselves to take a look around and see who else is lying on the floor beside us. Who else's life is falling apart? Who else is waiting and longing for something that is just beyond their reach?

This is the miraculous thing about being authentic in our trials of waiting. There is a community around us of people who are waiting, too. And if we let it, if we submit and lean on the Lord to give us wisdom to endure our trials as James says,[44] we become a community that reflects to the world the deep comfort of Christ. As we empathize, as we weep for others in a way that is comforting for them and comforting for us, as we endure and walk with them, the world sees the body of Christ as a healing place for the broken, not as an elite club.

I wonder if that's also why Christ suffered on our behalf—not just because the wages of sin is death, but also because we, too, need to see a suffering Savior. We need the community of His suffering. There is no weakness or shame in dependence. We were created as a body that is completely and solely sustained by the Head: Christ. We cannot carry our loads alone, nor are we ever meant to. Our waiting causes us to reach out to others because we need them. We cannot stand it any longer; we cannot stand on our own feet; we

---

44   James 1:2–7

reach out for comfort, and there we find each other. When the world catches a glimpse of how we care for one another in suffering, they get a glimpse of our Christ.

For Further Reflection

1. Have there been times you have sensed someone's pity more than their empathy? What was the difference?

2. Can you think of ways your own experiences have helped you offer empathy to others? How might they help you offer encouragement in the future?

3. What community have you found because of your waiting season?

4. Who might the Lord be leading you to empathize with in their journey of waiting, too? Who else is suffering around you?

5. How has your empathy and compassion toward others changed as you have endured your own sufferings and waiting on God?

CHAPTER FIFTEEN

What Waiting Does for Our Character

"But I will look to this one, At one who is humble and contrite in spirit, and who trembles at My word."

Isaiah 66:2

Waiting doesn't just affect our ability to relate with others. It also affects our character if we let it. Waiting strips us of pride and humbles us.

Humble Postures

Humility is not my favorite word. It is something we all say that we want, but we don't *really* want what it takes to get it. We want the outcome, not the work to achieve it. It is not a characteristic earned by striving or straining. It's not a popular topic like "leadership development" or "self-care." Humility is the smooth surface of wood that comes forth after being chafed against by coarse sandpaper. It is the soft surface of powdery sand underneath your feet, on a beach where pounding waves have worn shells down to granules. Everyone loves the beach and well-polished wood, but few of us welcome the realities that bring about such humility in our own lives.

The COVID-19 pandemic that started in 2020 is proof of this. The reality that we have no control—the reality that all our preparation, all our policies, all our thinking ahead did not protect us against this massive season of anxiety and catastrophe—humbled us in ways none of us would have chosen.

We don't welcome the circumstances, but they develop in us a healthy fear of the fact that we, ultimately, are not in control. They teach us humility.

I imagine the scene of Moses and the Israelites at the Red Sea. On one side was the thundering sound of horse hooves and chariots bearing down on them by the second. On the other was the engulfing sea, perhaps swollen and foaming. Pinned in the middle were Moses and the people God had just rescued from slavery. At that moment, it looked like they had been rescued only to be enslaved again. I can imagine the confusion, the wailing, and the fear swelling among the crowds. I can imagine them looking to Moses with panic on their faces as they quieted babies and reshuffled bags. In the agony, amid the assumption of defeat, Moses told the people to simply be still and wait on the Lord.[45]

How counterintuitive is that? Everyone around him would have been screaming, "Do something!" I will ever wonder how Moses would even be physically able to stay still in such a crisis. Maybe he was calm, but perhaps, he was shaking like a leaf. I imagine his heartbeat racing, his thoughts whirling, his whole body trembling as he stood perched on the edge of his ability and on the verge of God's deliverance.

Staying still when everyone around you is telling you to do something is more than a little challenging. Don't run around and try to make everything come together as it ought? Don't seek a way out of the waiting, the pain, the circumstances that are pinning me down? Don't look for a solution on my own? My tendency is not to sit in humility, welcoming the rescue from God's hand in His timing. That's a dreadfully uncomfortable place to be sometimes. When we are waiting for healing to come, for restoration in relationship, for clarity, for vision, for an opportunity to pursue our dreams, when we are waiting for God to arrive, it is uncomfortable. Everything in us and around us are screaming, "Do something!" We want to make something happen, make a way, forge ahead, keep moving. We are told, "God can't steer a parked car."

45 Exodus 14:10-21

Well, we do need to be ready to act, but often, we act without submitting to God's timing and way first.

I don't often wait for God to act, or trust Him to, because it leaves me in the position of having to be humble and admit that I don't have a way out. Humility is our true place, our only place in the cosmos. Yet we do not wear it willingly. It is often only *after* we have exhausted all that we can, *after* we have overturned every rock, that we admit the reality that was true at the very beginning of the search: He is in control. After all, how did Job respond after God questioned Him?[46] What complaint could Job offer to a God Who tells the sun to rise, maintains the earth's axis, and watches over everything else in the universe? He had to retract his complaint and repent in dust and ashes. Humility and submission are our only true place. Not that we are not valued or loved, but we have more limits than we like to think.

As a people, in the West we are very self-assured. We can remedy most situations with resources, information, knowledge, specialists, and money. We really believe we can do most things on our own, and to a degree, we can. The pandemic proved otherwise; it proved that we have less control than we wish to admit. Now I live in a place where people don't have savings, insurance companies, medicines and specialists, bail outs, or the security of all the things we think are important in the West. They live tied to the land and, in some ways, tied to the crises that befall it. This isn't the preferred state, let me tell you, but it has its merits. People here are much more willing to admit their humanity. They need and expect a lot of miracles. They depend on God in ways we believe are no longer necessary because of our financial means and self-actualization. But we know what will befall the proud. The Lord is close to the meek, to the broken-hearted, to those who know their need of Him.

Waiting can put us back into the place of humility that we ought to inhabit. It moves us from the position of lord to the position of servant.

46 Job 42:1-6

Waiting reminds us that we are the created, not the Creator. Humility and fear of the Lord are the beginnings of wisdom and trust. Humility leads us to beg for more of the Spirit of God to sustain us, lead us, and provide for us. Waiting is like thirst. It leads our souls to the Source of living water, our satiation, and reminds us that we are dependent rather than self-sufficient. Let it lead us to still waters to have our souls be restored, as we remember our identity as sheep in the loving fold of our Divine Shepherd.

Faithful Prayers

Behold, the eye of the LORD is on those who fear Him,

On those who wait for His faithfulness,

To rescue their soul from death

And to keep them alive in famine.

Our soul waits for the LORD;

He is our help and our shield.

For our heart rejoices in Him,

Because we trust in His holy name.

Let Your favor, LORD, be upon us,

Just as we have waited for You.

Psalm 33:18-22

The country in which my family and I are currently living, Malawi, is in desperate need of better healthcare. It has some of the worst health outcomes in the world. This is a place where people die from high blood pressure, malaria, or from asphyxia at birth. Death is so common, it is staggering. Our home country, Canada, has ambulances and emergency services, physicians and specialists, all forms of treatments and medications. We seek to make these services accessible to all, irrelevant of wealth or status. It's amazing and, comparatively, extravagant.

Here in the land in which we are living, the wealthy get better medical care, period. The suffering because of that reality is heart-wrenching. I cannot talk with someone for long without inevitably discussing a close family member, a child, or a husband who has died. That would make the news back in Canada, but here, it is unfortunately common. Imagine, lives lost because treatments are simply unavailable, or worse, they are available at a cost that you will never be able to afford—simple procedures and treatments.

It feels altogether criminal. It feels hopeless. Sometimes, I feel like I am drowning in the sadness of it all. I try to get up for air, only to pass by another funeral or hear of another person's loss. It feels so incredibly unjust when I consider from where I have come and to what we have access. I think about my children, and I can barely breathe if I consider losing them to something so incredibly basic, like a run-of-the-mill childhood illness. It's beyond painful to witness, let alone experience.

I was confused when I first arrived and met the Christian community here. They seem, well, rather intense and religious. They have all-night vigils, fast often and for long periods of time, and hold prayer meetings way more than I am used to. To be honest, I have never in my life gone to an all-night prayer vigil. I judged this community, at first. "Don't they know that they don't have to do that to be saved? Don't they know they can relax a bit?" I quickly realized the error of my judgments. That "religiosity" was not ritual religiosity at all. It was dependence. They are battling against the very reality of life here.

I suppose back in the West, we don't see the need to pray like this. Our immediate needs are often met. For the middle-class American or Canadian, we have clothes to wear, food to eat, and houses in which to live. Death and disease are the greatest burdens people face here in Malawi, and they know it. They pray because they are desperate for God's help. They expect great things from God, and He does them!

What else can you do when there is no money, access to healthcare, or reliable treatments, when life-saving medications may or may not be available, when transportation costs too much for people to get to a medical center, when practitioners might not even be trained to treat your illness? What else can you do but throw your hands up in the air, drop your knees onto the earth, and pray like you have never prayed before? And so it is, that we ought to be desperate for God's help in all things, at all times. Then I wonder, though they are monetarily poor, are they actually the rich? They realize their true state of dependency that we are blind to because of our wealth. This by no means negates their suffering, but it can help bring them to a closer relationship with God through the suffering.

Prayer—that thing that we say we do but don't really keep up with. Or, at least, that's my struggle. Do I pray—not out of religiosity, but out of complete dependency?

The other day, my youngest daughter, barely three, became very sick. I cannot tell you the fear that gripped my heart. We could not find a trusted practitioner; no one could tell us what was going on; and I was worried like I have never been before. I can't "wait and see" what will happen, like I am accustomed to in Canada. If we "wait and see," it might be too late to get where we need to go to help her recover. A simple and basic illness, and I am flat on the ground, bawling off my face, praying for God's help. I love this dear girl so terribly much that I cannot help but fear the worst.

To lose her would be like losing myself. She has been, in every way, God's gift to me. What if we cannot get her the medical help she needs? A friend said, "It's like living by the skin of your teeth here." I'm not sure that statement comforted me as much as it threw me into a panic. We are the ones, her parents, who have knowingly chosen to live in this place of inadequate healthcare to help with that exact problem. Yet could I ever forgive myself if something happened to my children as a result?

Desperation—we don't like to let ourselves experience it. We have so many plan B's and ways to buy ourselves out of problems that we rarely get to the point of desperation. We can pull out the credit card, get on the internet, cash in a favor, or manipulate and navigate our way through most circumstances without so much as a holler upstairs toward God's throne. We have house insurance and bank accounts and refrigerators. We so rarely have to feel the magnitude of desperation that I sense my neighbors in this country carry with them every day. The line between eating and starving is so thin; the glass between kids attending and not attending school is so transparent; the film between health and death is so fragile.

To have to wait on God for some areas of our lives is a gift to us in many ways that we probably fail to realize. When we think of the thing for which we are waiting on God, we have to cry out to Him and recognize our own helplessness. In this part of our lives, at least, we are reminded from where our help truly comes and embrace our complete and utter dependence on Him. This can lead us toward faithfulness to Him, if we let it. We ought to be banging His door down as we cry out to Him. We ought to be having prayer vigils and fasting and asking and seeking and knocking. We ought to be going to Him, our very Source of life and breath, instead of running around opening every other door.

I know this has been true in my life. In the hardest places of my greatest desperation, I have worn down a smooth path on the pavement where I have cried out to God. Not because begging is what gets God's attention but because our hearts need to be reminded of on Whom we should depend.

You might think that you are waiting on God to come through or respond, but maybe He's actually the One waiting on you. He's waiting for you to cry out to Him, waiting for you to trust Him, waiting for you to look to Him, waiting for you to lean on Him in new ways. Maybe it's time to recognize your complete and utter dependence, to faithfully arrive at His throne, and to continue asking for the thing your heart desires. Maybe it's time to pray like you have never prayed. We like to think we have prayed; but often, we have talked about prayer and asked people to pray for us, but we ourselves have not really offered our requests to God.

Persevering Hearts

Blessed is a man who perseveres under trial; for once he has been approved, he will receive the crown of life which the Lord has promised to those who love Him.

James 1:12

When James, the brother of Christ, was writing his letter (the book of James) to the scattered Christians abroad, what did he mean by trials? We think about the persecution and poverty they were facing, the rejection by their peers, and for some, their martyrdom. We know that when James was writing about trials, he meant those trials. But as we study this passage, we know that he also meant trials of various kinds that afflict and will continue to afflict us as we walk on this earth. There will be hardships, diseases, losses, injustices, and the list goes on and on. Satan is bound and determined to get at us in any way he can. Many of these trials (or sometimes referred to as temptations) will test us. God uses them in our lives to strengthen and develop our character. Without trials and difficulties, we cannot become "perfect and complete, lacking in nothing" (James 1:4).

What is meant by the testing of our faith? Imagine a chair. That chair could represent our faith. Every trial we face has a weight to it—a weight of pain, sorrow, grief—a weight that is heavy and hard to carry on our own. But our faith in God is like that chair. Chairs are of no use just sitting there empty. Faith is of no use if it is in our minds but affects nothing about the way we live. To test out a chair is to sit in the chair. To test our faith is to put the weight of trials onto our faith. Will our faith hold up underneath the trials? Will it stand solid and firm, not moved or crushed by the heaviness of the circumstances in which we find ourselves? Or will our faith collapse under the weight of our trials?

I used to imagine the word *testing* differently—maybe like an obstacle course or an academic test. The aim of these tests is to prove yourself by what you know or are capable of doing. But that's not what is meant here. To withstand the test of trials, our faith must endure; bear under the weight of our pain; and bravely, courageously, and trustingly remain faithful to God no matter what may come. Will I trust Him even when it all falls apart?

We are never asked to hold up under the weight of our trials on our own. Jesus says we are to take heart, since He has overcome the world.[47] He says He will never abandon us.[48] He says that we are to come to Him when we are in need of rest.[49] He says His "burden is light."[50] He says to be still, to not fear, and to take courage because of His presence with us.[51]

Waiting times are trials. They are painful; they are wearying; they are frustrating. Waiting to get papers to move countries, waiting for autism diagnoses, waiting for political change, waiting to get into medical school— there are so many seasons in which we find ourselves waiting. But they are trials put in our path to endure faithfully. They are exactly what James is talking about. They can test our faith. They bear a weight. When that pressure of time is added onto the load, how will we choose to respond?

The word for trial in some translations is "temptation." Every trial is an opportunity to be strengthened in our faith and resolve to believe God for Who He says He is and is also a temptation to walk away, to disbelieve God, to give way to the weight of our hardships and question the only One able to help us bear up underneath them.

We live in a world that lacks endurance. At the first sign of hardship, we often run and flee. We might physically escape our trials, or we escape emotionally.

---

47   John 16:33
48   Hebrews 13:5
49   Matthew 11:28
50   Matthew 11:30
51   Deuteronomy 31:6

We seal ourselves off; we disconnect; we hide away; we numb ourselves; we do anything we can to isolate the pain and disassociate from it. Nobody likes to be uncomfortable, and we live in a world where ease is the prize. We look for an easier way, a faster way, a satisfying way. But it's deceptive. What one gains in temporary reprieve, one loses in character growth and development. What one gains in momentary escape, one loses in endurance. There is no way around it, only through it. You cannot strengthen weak muscles without applying pressure, weight, and stress on them. And weak muscles of faith will tear and sprain if not tested under the weight of affliction. Muscles will not grow without resistance, and neither will our faith.

I have always adored hydrangeas in Canada, a beautiful bush that grows large balls of purple, blue, or white flowers. The hue is determined by the soil's acidity. As a dreamy teenager, I used to wander neighborhoods, gazing with wonder at all the shades of purple, finding ways to sneak a few balls from the bushes to bring them home to dry. As an adult, my dream was to have one in my garden. Early one spring, I bought my first potted hydrangea and decided to mother it until it was time to transplant it outside. I thought it would be easy to transfer it outside, and being a novice gardener, I did just that. I didn't think about having to make the plant hardier to endure being outside.

Of course, it died because I didn't know how much time and patience was required. I didn't know that I needed to move it inside and outside repetitively so that it could grow in endurance. I didn't know that I had to give it enough time to withstand the wind, the rain, the sun, or any of the other elements in order to prepare it to survive. I had left it housebound and in an environment of relative ease. It had no strength, no character, no ability to withstand the realities of the wild. I wasn't willing to let my hydrangea go through that kind of process, and in the end, I lost out from the beauty and life it could have produced every year if I had done just that.

If a hydrangea with a loving, careful, and knowledgeable caretaker had thoughts, it might question why it was being shut outdoors for periods of time, while its owner watched from ease and comfort behind glass windows. Being battered and bruised by wind and rain, it would wonder how it could possibly be abandoned in the great outdoors. But ultimately, it wouldn't have to wonder because the very beauty it would produce, though at a cost to its comfort, would demonstrate reason enough for the plight it endured.

Isn't that what we want—to flourish and bring beauty? How easy it is to bend and break beneath the weight of our sorrows and trials. How easy it is to slip into despair and bow down to fear and envy. How easy it is to crumble and fall into self-pity and to question God's goodness. But waiting upon God for strength and comfort will achieve for us a greater glory than we can possibly imagine. Accepting hardship willingly, for the joy of enduring until the end, is not the world's way. But it is God's way. And to think that God could take the broken, shattered pieces of our lives, the stretched-thin and worn-down places, and turn them into something beautiful that brings Him glory is way better than what the world has to offer. "For our momentary, light affliction is producing for us an eternal weight of glory far beyond all comparison, while we look not at the things which are seen, but at the things which are not seen; for the things which are seen are temporal, but the things which are not seen are eternal" (2 Cor. 4:17-18).

The "small" troubles you are facing probably do not feel small. Waiting does not feel small. It feels all-encompassing. If your world feels like it is breaking and shifting, if you feel like you are beyond your ability to withstand the pain of it, that's exactly where God shows up.

The truth is that it *is* beyond you. The world so often tells us to be more independent, to show grit and courage, to pull ourselves up by our bootstraps and be capable. But Jesus, perfect in strength and holiness, still came before His Father on the night He was betrayed and wept so hard that there was blood.[52] He modeled complete surrender and complete dependence. We are not created to walk this alone. We are incapable, in our own strength, to

---

52 Luke 22:39-46

continue walking in our trials. We are in desperate need of help and courage. Some days, we will feel like we can climb mountains. God will give us peace and joy amid our greatest sorrows. Other days, we will be a wreck on the floor, wondering how we will possibly make it through another minute or hour of waiting for reprieve. But the grace is that we have only this moment in which to walk. We can face this one with His hand in ours. We don't have to face our whole lives in one minute or hour. We just have to face the next moment. And that we can do when we know that God will not let us be pulled under the waves and can save us from total despair.

There were many days when the thought of death was easier than the thought of enduring another night without sleep. The thought of days, upon months, upon years of my life until the bitter end filled without sleep was incomprehensible. These endless days were like the giants in the land that the Israelites spied. They looked insurmountable.[53]

If we focus on our giants, life is impossible. But if we focus on our God, it's possible. This isn't just a platitude. Our gaze determines our direction. If we gaze on our troubles, on a future full of them, we simply cannot stand. We have to look to our God, Who is not only able to save us *from* our waiting but save us *in* the waiting. He will give us mature faith and perseverant hearts in the middle of it.

For Further Reflection

1. How do you see your character growing and changing through your trial of waiting?
2. What do you think God might be trying to teach you?
3. How are you experiencing His presence *with* you today?
4. What steps can you take to talk to God more freely and honestly? Commit to a weekend of prayer, a time of fasting and prayer, or a prayer journal.

---

53 Numbers 13:26-30

CHAPTER SIXTEEN

What Waiting Does in Our Relationship with God

But as for me, the nearness of God is good for me;

I have made the Lord God my refuge,

So that I may tell of all Your works.

Psalm 73:28

Have you ever been led through a room blindfolded like my experience at the Dark Table? What is the best way for someone to lead you? Sure, they could give you verbal directions. They could say, "Go right; go left; look out!" But inevitably, you would probably run into something. It's not the best method to keep you safe because your interpretation of what they say might not match what they intended. How big of a step did they mean? How far right? Turn abruptly or just slightly to the right? Of course, you would end up taking teeny, tiny baby steps, moving forward as slow as molasses to avoid the dangerous possibilities resulting from misinterpreting their words.

How different the experience is when someone takes you by the hand or when you put your hand on their shoulder and they lead you through the room. The risk becomes theirs, not yours. When they are right in front of you, if they make an error in judgment and bump into something, they will be hurt, not you. You can move much faster, too, with this method. If you trust the person with whom you are physically in contact, you can walk swiftly through a crowd even without so much as bumping into someone.

His Presence

I wonder about what it means to walk through the dark times in our lives holding on to God's presence. What if we believed that He did, in fact, have us in His grip during our darkest seasons? What if we believed that we could not stumble or fall or go the wrong way while sticking with Him? What if we believed He was that Sovereign?

I have heard enough stories of suffering and sadness in my profession to know that something happens in suffering that is different from other times in our lives. Pretense collapses. We are left with what is at the very core. On what rock are we found standing? If we are followers of Jesus and looking to Him, He will lead us in the dark, but not as a distant Voice we have to strain our ears to hear. He will lead us by His very touch, by His very presence. His grace becomes palpable. His touch penetrates the longest, darkest nights of our lives and consoles in ways beyond what it does in the light.

When someone bears witness to another person's suffering, they often are found saying, "I just don't know how they are surviving this. I don't know that I could do it." I believe God gives special grace to us in our difficult seasons if we ask Him for it. I have seen many people weather storms in their lives that I cannot stand the thought of having to bear—the sudden death of a spouse or child, the trauma of a family member dealing with mental health struggles, divorce, loss of job and home, and more. For those who have an active and living faith, I have marveled on the sidelines as they have weathered these storms with otherworldly grace and peace. From the outside I cannot *understand* how they are managing because I am not in their shoes. But when we face these sorts of trials, there is grace available to us in them. When we ask, He is there in ways we may have never before experienced. He is the Eye of the storm, the Center of peace when everything spins around us.

This is true of our waiting seasons, too. I don't know what it feels like waiting for a wayward child to come home. I don't know what it feels like to wait for a spouse after years of searching. I don't know what it feels like to wait for so many things, but I do know there is grace available to each of us in our unique trials of waiting.

There are many passages about the Lord's nearness to those who call on Him. He is not a God Who is far off. The very hope of the Gospel lies in the fact that God chose to come near to us. Dark seasons in our lives don't mean the absence of His presence. Just because our situation has gone from bad to worse doesn't mean He is farther away. Maybe we don't understand what He is doing. Maybe we feel abandoned. Maybe we are in that dark room and cannot see Him, but He has not left us in it. As the psalmist says, "The LORD is near to all who call on Him, To all who call on Him in truth" (Psalm 145:18).

As we call out to Him in the dark, He will answer. Even when no one else can comfort, when no one else can restore our spirits, when our eyes are raw from crying, God comes near when we call to Him. And from His lips comes, "'Do not fear!'" (Lamentations 3:57). He will guide us. We may be afraid as we reach out our hands and close our eyes, but we can be assured that His nearness will be our strength. Where we cannot see, He will walk before us and lead us in the way everlasting.

Stop looking for the light under doorways, straining your eyes for the dawn, and flipping on your cellphone to light your path. He *is* your Light. Lean on Him and let Him guide you, for He is the One Who created light itself.

I know what it is like to live in the darkness of waiting and to feel the apparent absence of God. In the stumbling, wandering, painful early years of motherhood as I tried to carry on without sleep and insomnia dragged me to the end of myself, I had many choices to make. I often didn't make the right ones. I often ran from God and tried to solve my own issue. I didn't recognize I was choosing my own way instead of God's presence. I often nurtured my own distrust and grew in bitterness, thinking God was choosing to be far off. But how could I experience His nearness when I was too busy panicking and trying to find a way out of the mess? It was only in stillness, in a crumpled heap of tears, that I was able to finally recognize His grace in the whispers, songs, and moments of His presence. He *was* there, but I was neglecting to see Him.

My second son was born into this fiery trial; and maybe to console me, or maybe as a declaration, we named him Tobin Emmanuel. Tobin means "God is good." Somehow in the depth of my despair, He revealed His goodness and His nearness to me, not in the answer to my suffering but amid it. Emmanuel means "God is with us." When all I could see was my own despair, the horizon from my view was dotted with endless sleepless nights, and I was being unraveled completely, knowing He was with me in it was enough of a comfort to get through the night. Even if I had to shout it to the darkness, scream it at the top of my lungs so that I could hear myself above my own panic, I would declare it, nonetheless.

Our Submission

The mountains melted like wax at the presence of the LORD,

At the presence of the LORD of the whole earth.

The heavens declare His righteousness,

And all the peoples have seen His glory.

Psalm 97:5-6

Another way we fail to acknowledge the activity of God in our lives is in our quest for control. In our relationship with God, we grow comfortably detached from His Lordship. Though we know God is with us, we often live as if He were not. To the core of who we are as broken, sinful people is a desire to be masters over ourselves. To not have control and mastery is what we consider slavery. Slavery is a difficult subject; it is the antithesis of all the Western world values, yet an unfortunate reality in our history—consequences of which are still felt today. Self-determination is rightfully desired rather than enslavement. To not have the ability to live, work, or do anything of one's own choice or out from beneath the oppression of others is unjust. To be enslaved is to have one's freedom forcibly removed. We have seen this play out in history and continue to work to rid society of the effects of systemic oppression, but how do we also interact with the opposite concept, that of freedom, in our daily personal lives?

We as humans adore the idea of individual freedom—freedom from obligation to family, culture or gender, obligation to government, obligation to constructs and institutions, and freedom from Divine authority.

Though we value social efforts to provide opportunities and freedom, this word "freedom" is a bit of an illusion. We are never completely free. There are always natural limits and consequences to our actions. If we reject boundaries and constructs, rules and rhythms, we inevitably face other subjugation. Maybe we have the choice to be whomever we want to be and work hard for that goal. But as we choose to live limitless, productive, achieving, social-climbing lives, we end up with anxiety and stress on our bodies and declining health as we pursue an ever-moving line of "enough" achievement. Is that freedom?

Maybe we have the freedom to choose to use drugs and alcohol at our own discretion, but what happens if numbing becomes our only means of surviving our daily life? What happens when our flesh cannot be controlled? We become slaves to our substances. Maybe we have the freedom to use any and all technology to connect and be entertained, but what happens when we can no longer put away the phone or turn off the social media feeds, and we become tyrannized by fear and anxiety because of all the opinions and fear-mongering? The Bible is clear that we are terrible masters of our own lives. The desires of our broken selves—and the prideful belief that we have the strength to tame our sinful and backward flesh on our own—make us unwilling to submit ourselves to our heavenly Father. We are free to choose Him or not, but make no mistake, choosing to command our own flesh without the help of His Spirit is futile in every way.

Oh, but we like to think and believe we are able. We like to believe that we have complete control over our lives. If we just work harder, plan better, have more, be smarter, then we will have the life we want. However, is that really true? An earthquake hits; a car accident happens; economies crash; one tiny virus arrives; the list goes on. Just when we start outsmarting the world and our biology (or so we think), we get a slap in the face and realize we actually have little real control. It's traumatic when we have to recognize that for all of the good intentions, planning, and providing for ourselves, we actually cannot predict or control our lives.

But what does it mean to surrender and submit to God as the Master of our lives? What does it mean to readily and freely live under His Lordship? He is not a tyrant. He is a loving Father and to submit to His Lordship *is* true freedom.

I know a lot about one form of surrender; I see it every day when patients step into a hospital. Before entering the hospital, they were just any other person on the street. They might have been shoulder to shoulder with a nurse or doctor on the bus, and there would be no vulnerability or submission between the two strangers. But as this person enters a hospital, there is an implicit expectation that they are willing to submit themselves to the care, knowledge, and competency of their healthcare providers. Of course, nursing theory reiterates that a person's health is a mutual and shared responsibility, but there is still some submission required. There is a necessary vulnerability, a trust, as a person rolls up their sleeve for a blood pressure reading, as they stick out their arm for blood to be taken, or when they lie still as their lungs are listened to with a stethoscope. If they don't submit their body for assessment and observation, or present themselves for testing or examination, or don't agree to treatment plans, how can they expect to recover?

Submission is not a word we value in our society. The idea that one's rights should willingly be laid down for another person is unpopular. Submission is an action, a verb that means accepting or yielding to the will or authority of another. As parents of children, we know that we often must submit our bodies, our time, and our attention to someone else, even when we don't feel like it. As spouses, we may yield our desires to allow our spouse to pursue their dreams; and they may do the same for us. As friends, we are willing to give up our time to help others, to offer ourselves and our resources to them because love demands that we do.

Of course, submission is easy when there's something in it for me, when something is given in return for that submission. It's easy to think about our losses when we give ourselves to God. But when we submit our will, our desires, our hopes, our dreams, our plans, our bodies, and our very lives to the living God, we get more than we ever lose.

In times of waiting and longing, to willingly offer our hopes to God is a choice. He will not force us to make it—as discussed earlier, forced submission is just slavery—but circumstances might encourage us to do so. Waiting times teach us that it's preposterous, even impossible, to receive His loving care without surrender. Do we trust Him like we trust our physicians? Do we roll up our sleeves, hand in our street clothes, and trust that He knows what is best for us better than we do? Do we entrust our dreams to Him? Do we entrust our children? Do we entrust our work, our purpose, our careers, our every aspect of life to Him? This will never feel "natural." This will never feel "comfortable."

We are told and believe that we have rights to our life and our own decisions, but God's kingdom is upside down. He had rights to Heaven, yet He chose to come to earth and give everything up to save us. Will we follow Christ's lead and entrust our lives to our Father for His glory and our good?

Becoming More Present to Our Actual Lives

After you have suffered for a little while, the God of all grace, who called you to His eternal glory in Christ, will Himself perfect, confirm, strengthen, and establish you.

1 Peter 5:10

My husband often laughs at my propensity to fast-walk. Whenever I was pregnant, he would often express relief at me being physically unable to walk my usual "tail-on-fire" speed. I'd glare at him and remind him that one day, we'd walk our usual way—me at least twenty feet ahead of him. Funnily enough, I've never thought it odd that I am not literally walking *with* my husband when we go on walks *together*. Somehow, I still feel like we are on a walk together, even if I am a hundred meters ahead.

I don't know what it is, but I simply cannot stand moving slowly. I blame it on my short stature, which has always meant I have to take one extra step to keep up with everyone else's long-legged strides. I blame my fast-walking pace on my height but also on my crazy nursing career, which demands that I run for twelve hours at a time. Ultimately, however, it's part of my personality. I simply don't like dawdling. I can't stand riding escalators, especially if people don't follow the rules and stay to the right if standing. I am, obviously, never the one standing. I'm competitive and a little too proud of my ability to multitask and accomplish a lot in short periods of time. So, I figure if I just move faster, I'll get everything done faster. I'm not saying it's the better way, either, because in my rushing, I inevitably spill more, break more glassware, get in more fender benders, and miss critical steps for which I simply do not take the time.

It is no surprise, then, that I have been gifted with a little boy who sees life in a very different way. This kid dawdles like his life depends on it. The combination of the two of us has always been quite a scene. I remember school pick-up time years ago: I was off and running to get to the car so that we could avoid the inevitable after-school traffic jam, dragging my toddler in one hand and carrying the baby in another, dodging crowds like it was a competitive sport. And there was my five-year-old son, inching along a hundred feet or more behind. Sometimes, I literally forgot that he was behind me, and I spent more time than I ought shouting, "Hurrrrrry up!" I huffed and puffed, sighed, rolled my eyes, cajoled, harped, nagged, threatened being hit by cars, and displayed any number of uttered frustrations at this unfortunate difference in our paces.

He is slow about pretty much everything. Even still, as a nine-year-old, he lines his shoes up meticulously while I throw mine across the room and aim for the shoe bench. He takes twenty-five-minute bathroom trips, while I sometimes time myself to see if I can beat my record for speed. He eats dinner like he's at a five-star restaurant and needs to savor every bite, while I barely remember chewing and have already cleared the table and washed all the dishes before his plate is clean. His pace is a blessing to me—and a cause of great frustration. He is fully immersed in the right-now moments of his life, while I all too easily race past them.

When it comes to the uncomfortable seasons of our lives, the ones which we cannot wait to leave behind, we come to find that there is no rushing through them. We are so used to going about our lives at breakneck speeds—planning months in advance for trips, weeks in advance for friend-dates, and days in advance for errands—that we are unaccustomed to being present in all the everyday moments of our lives. The year of 2020 did a lot to change our recognition of how that kind of pace has been wreaking havoc on our mental health. But we still often are oblivious to the moments that should catch our breath with their beauty, that should cause us to worship in awe and wonder. We breeze past it all because we are too busy with our programs and productivity.

Then suddenly, we are thrust into a season of waiting, and it's like the time is frozen on the clock. Waiting for a vaccine, waiting for borders to open, waiting for governmental aid, waiting for social gatherings to be allowed, and waiting for the world to return to some sense of normal. It's maddening, really—like going from running on the pavement to running in wet cement.

I wonder, though, if that, too, is a lesson for us to be right here, right now, in the moments of our lives, to stop looking for what could be and settle into what is. Instead of looking ahead to the next intersection, the next freeway on-ramp, how can we better enjoy the view out our windows on this causeway? There have been far too many seasons of my life I have rushed by, only to realize I cannot relive them and savor them like I should have. I was so eager to get on to the next thing that I didn't appreciate that season for what it was—a small sliver of time in the length of my life. We sometimes get so deep into a season that we cannot see past it, but it will pass. We cannot see in the moment that it may be a sweet season—a period of preparation, a time of reflection, of growth and transformation—or, perhaps, a season we are meant to experience so that we are better prepared to enjoy the one ahead.

I never willingly enter seasons of slowness. Slow feels backward. Slow feels unproductive. Slow feels valueless. For so many years, I have prided myself on fast-paced multitasking, striving to accomplish and prove myself, and on building a life under my own control.

That first time I got sideswiped was through my knee injury. I was in my early twenties, and I simply did not know what to do. Every movement and action was impossible on an unstable joint. All of a sudden, amid making plans, running errands, finishing this project, meeting with that person, and living at breakneck speeds, I was flat on my back with my leg in the air. Nothing had prepared me to live on my back. What I imagined I could bounce back from became days and weeks and months of slow recovery. Learning how to walk again, bracing myself against doorways, grimacing at downhill gradients, sitting on the couch, and saying no to events became my way of life.

It is a strange experience to be part of the blur of life and then be sequestered to a bed, watching it all happen slowly around you. Suddenly, you are left with endless minutes of freedom—freedom to notice small changes in the world around you as you sit and watch time pass: the movement of a leaf on a tree, the specks of dust in the stream of sunlight, the way that fern arches just so.

At our home in Canada, I had a window in my bedroom that peered into our backyard. We had a few big trees in our yard, one of which was a large maple. We were told when we moved in that we should probably take it down.

We were told it was too large and that its root system would start to break apart the foundation of our home. However, my husband and I could not part with it. Its leaves were the size of our toddler's head and filled up the yard with their beautiful, light green hue all summer long. It provided shade, and the beauty of its colors as the leaves changed in fall was stunning. After my fourth C-section, I spent hours watching those leaves blow in the breeze. I spent time watching squirrels race along our fence's edge and the weather change while I nursed a newborn and looked out that window. It was life to me. I was surprised by how much joy I could find looking out the window.

I didn't easily weather those early years of being slowed down. But after my fourth baby, the slowness was life-giving to me. To have a serious excuse to stare at walls was a relief amid a busy household. I did not ask for or choose another surgery, believe me, but I appreciated the slowness of life it gifted me in a way I hadn't before. I reveled in looking out my window. What might I see today? What shadow would catch my attention? What bird might I spot?

Maybe waiting does this in us if we lean into it. When we stop fighting it, when we realize we cannot get what we long for *right now*, when all our energy wanes from striving after that which we have no control to obtain and we let go into the abyss of slow-moving time, do we start to see what's right in front of us? In our relationship with God, there is so much more available to us in this moment, but we often miss it.

We spend so much of our lives working for things and trying to gain control, but when we let go for God's plans, we are left with open space. That's when the stillness beckons in a new way. Suddenly, our hearts are free to embrace the moments of our everyday lives. When all the noise of planning and dreaming ends like a freight train against a wall and we are looking at a bunch of broken pieces, we simply sit among them and start looking around.

If we let it do its good work in us, waiting can give us the gift of seeing. In the dark, we can't see much. In fact, in the pitch black, we might not be able to see anything at all. But there are other senses God has gifted us. What a gift for the blind person to hear and feel and notice things that we might never notice. They feel things differently, hear things differently, and altogether experience the world differently because they are in tune to senses we sighted people are not. How much do we miss because of our sight?

In the same way, I wonder at all the things we miss because we are so busy figuring out everything, planning and strategizing our way out of hardship and grief and trials. We don't like to sit in hard times; we like to blow past them. We don't like to consider that waiting might be God's gift to us. We don't like to think that we could be missing valuable things in life because of impatience. But maybe life was meant to be richer on account of these periods of waiting. Maybe we would appreciate other seasons of our lives more fully because of them. Perhaps what we really need is to be present to our current circumstances and embrace them for what a gift they are.

Eternal Perspective

Therefore the Lord longs to be gracious to you,
And therefore He waits on high to have compassion on you.
For the Lord is a God of justice;
How blessed are all those who long for Him.

Isaiah 30:18

Ten years ago was the first time we lived in Africa. Orange dust filled our nostrils, blew in through the windows, and covered everything. Not a day went by when I didn't have to wash my counters and floors from the thick layer of dryness. All my clothes were permanently stained. To say that the climate was arid would be an understatement.

We were living in a small town, hundreds of miles from the capital city of one of the poorest countries in the world. It was a hot, dry, and water-impoverished landscape. The village we called home for just a short time was better known as "the place no one wanted to live." Even locals didn't want to move from the city to this rural area. No electricity, no running water, few amenities, and all the calamities that accompany such poverty of convenience.

But the one thing this place had in abundance was mango trees. They were everywhere. Coming from the Pacific coast where it's green year-round, the dry landscape held a beauty and mystery of which I never tired. But I appreciated those towering, green mango trees. They provided shade from the sweltering heat. In mango season, they were the center of village life. Children would climb their thick branches and shake down their fruit. I still remember the sound they made hitting the dry, water-starved ground.

After months of dry season, without a drop of rain, when all other crops had failed for lack of water, the mango trees would not shrivel up. It was at the end of the dry season that they would bear fruit. It was at the end of the dust storms and when the earth's crust started to crack from want of water that this tree would erupt in sweet and sticky fruit—thick, heavy, rich, sweet, and juicy fruit in abundance. People would sink not just their dusty lips into them but also their whole faces. Never have I tasted such a thing as fresh mangoes.

I marvel at the truth this represents to me. In a desert where it takes numerous attempts to sink a well, God, in His incomprehensible wisdom, provides water-rich fruit against all odds. And not just after the rains have descended upon the earth, but before—at the end of a long season of waiting. And in the way that only He can do, He brings life from nothing, fruit from parched land. In just the right season, in just the right time, when all who depend on its fruit are desperate for hope, the fruit comes.

I have seen what it means to live off the land as a subsistence farmer—how much they hold their breath and clasp hands together in prayer to whomever might listen. The very lives of their children hinge on whatever comes down from the sky and up from the ground. Without rain, there is no food. Without water, there is no life.

Here I sit, on the dry earth of my dreams, on my unfulfilled desires. It seems impossible that any life can come out of this dry ground. But I have hope that is creeping, budding, blooming in the midst of my dried-up dreams of an unmedicated sleep. What if the fruition of dreams comes not in the midst of triumphal rains, but after seasons of drought? What if God uses those seasons even more than we could imagine? It's been so long since I have felt the sky break and the sweet relief of answered prayers come pouring down on me. Arms stretched toward the heavens like the lonely mango tree branches, will I see the supernatural answer from the Divine? Will I await the realization of my hopes with a sure trust that God, in His perfect timing, will bring good fruit when the season is right?

It looks impossible. It feels treacherous at times, this waiting. But maybe waiting for the Supernatural to breathe life into the dust is actually the best place to be—where I stop trying to make the fruit come of my own strength but have to wait on God to do what only He can do—bring mangoes from the dust. How much louder our praise when His answer does come? How much greater glory does He receive? I want to sink my face into the miraculous provision from the hand of God. I want His sticky, sloppy provisions to drip off my cheeks while songs of praise and thanksgiving burst from my lips. There is nothing richer, nothing more beautiful than His miraculous supply.

So, while my bare feet wait on the dusty dirt and with my face to the skies, all my hope is in God, the only One Who can bring fruit from dust, the only One Who can take my humble, dusty dreams and bring them to life.

For Further Reflection

1. What are some "mangoes" in your life? Where have you seen God's miraculous provision at the end of a season of waiting?

2. How can you practice gratitude and praise in this time of waiting?

3. How is your personal relationship with God? In what ways has He already demonstrated His grace, His kindness, and His proximity to your suffering?

4. What changes can you make to draw closer to the One Who is sitting in your dark night with you?

5. What world events have taught you about your lack of control? In what areas do you need to loosen your own grip?

6. In the stillness of your season of waiting, what is right in front of you that you have been too busy running past to notice?

7. How present are you to God, people, and the natural beauty around you? How has this season of waiting in your life made you more present to other neglected parts of your life?

Final Thoughts

Come, let's sing for joy to the Lord,

Let's shout joyfully to the rock of our salvation.

Let's come before His presence with a song of thanksgiving,

Let's shout joyfully to Him in songs with instruments.

For the Lord is a great God

And a great King above all gods,

In whose hand are the depths of the earth,

The peaks of the mountains are also His.

The sea is His, for it was He who made it,

And His hands formed the dry land.

Come, let's worship and bow down,

Let's kneel before the Lord our Maker.

For He is our God.

Psalm 95:1-7

I am staring out as the sun sets, lost in thought. I am thinking about things for which I long, feeling the ache of them—places I long to see, things I long to do. One longing bleeds into another one like watercolors. Then I think about what I have spent most of my life waiting for.

The Waiting

For years, my husband and I dreamed of a life overseas. We are adventurers, explorers, learners, and laborers. We knew in our hearts, from early in our marriage, that we were destined to go abroad. But there we were, eleven years and many twists and turns later, still in Canada. "Here" became synonymous with "settling." I never wanted to settle. In fact, if you could ask my seventeen-year-old self what I feared the most in life, I would have said, "Settling." I have always been addicted to change and disruption. The idea of doing anything that was in any way ordinary felt like a cursed life. I know that is, in fact, some individual's ideal life, but I never wanted that. Settling was not who I was.

Yet it had been eleven years, and settled we were. We were "here" when I wanted to be "there." Obviously, there are still lessons for me to learn about contentment and being *in* the seasons to which God has called me, but despite our attempts to do what we felt "called to," we still hit every closed door. I mean, *every* closed door.

Health problems kept us "here." Fear of taking risks kept us "here." Uncertainty and lack of clarity kept us "here." Ultimately, God kept us "here."

I started out angry. Then I threw blame like bullets. I did a whole lot of envying and a bucketload of comparing, and there were emotions flying around like pollen on a spring day. Then came the strategizing and reorganizing, the planning and recalculating. The cerebral me jumped right in for a kick at the can. "If I just manipulate this that way and if I just coerce and control, then I'll get my dream come true." But when reality set in that this particular waiting season—a separate journey of waiting from my insomnia—was here to stay, that's when things got really ugly.

I was heartsick. That's when I started cutting people out who had what I wanted—avoiding, dulling the pain, running away from responsibility, dreaming of higher hills and greener pastures without Him at the reins. In some frantic last effort, my flesh grabbed at anything I could to avoid this stretched-thin feeling of waiting.

What does waiting feel like? It feels like sadness. It feels like loss. It feels heavy and relentless. It feels lonely and aching. It feels hollow and empty.

My knee-jerk reaction to waiting has been anything but beautiful. Turns out, when I try to get through the waiting on my terms, it ends up looking a lot like striving, a lot like bitterness and manipulation, and gets me no nearer to the vision for which I hoped.

Yet all along, God's voice was inviting me into the silence, into the stillness, and into the void of waiting. When I put down my frantic calculating and emotional posturing, His voice invited me to sit. His is a Voice that does not carry panic or frustration. It doesn't accuse and tell me, "You're not good enough, prove you can do it!" or "You're running out of time!" No, His voice invites me into something altogether different.

God's voice invites me to calm down. Trust. Believe in His goodness. Believe in His sovereignty. Believe in His timing. To be honest, even though I now sit overseas while I write this, exactly where I hoped I might be, do you think I am satisfied? Or do you think I have walked right into another season of waiting? It's not been a perfect ending; it comes with its own pains and longings. While one hope and dream might be neatly tidied up, in some ways there are still a thousand questions that remain. Behind the door to the land of "there" was a new set of yearnings.

"What next? What then? What now?" On and on the questions go. The greatest lie I ever believed was that there was such a thing as "arrival" on this side of Heaven. One question leads down a rabbit hole to a thousand more, and I find myself in new seasons of waiting for other things. Contentment is hard-earned on this finite earth of mystery and fog.

"There is a richness to the learning curve of not running ahead of Him." These words were spoken over me before this last waiting time, and I chafed against them like new shoes on bare heels. But they are settling down to the center of me and bubbling up and out, like an overflowing spring. It is, indeed, a learning curve to which I continue to have to adjust with each new trial of waiting.

Will I accept only the plateaus and not the valleys from Him? The landscape of our lives would be devoid of beauty if there were no depths. Heights are only heights because of the great surrounding valleys that enhance the vistas. If we always got what we wanted, if we never had to wait, if there was no yearning or needing or longing, what space would our lives hold for God? He is the Author of our waiting, as much as He is the Author of our receiving. Sometimes, I wonder if our waiting space is simply Him carving out space for Himself in our souls. Will we go to Him in our need and hold out our hands, not afraid to ask and want and need more of Him? After all, the kingdom of God is for the needy and the poor, the sick and the blind, those who have not and who come to Him requesting and looking for all that they lack. He tells us to come if we are weary, and He will give us rest. But will we be drawn by the shadows and holes in our lives or repelled?

No one wants to settle for the semi-good ending—one where the dream is half-realized. I don't want to settle for my own rendition of how I think my life should go. But I have to say, there's a lot more waiting in this life than I ever thought there'd be. And sometimes, staying "here" to wait for Him to bring me "there" looks a lot more like obedience than I thought. It looks a lot more active, too—choosing to be thankful, choosing joy, choosing trust, choosing to enter into relationships, even through my grimaced face and wet cheeks. It looks like choosing to celebrate those who get to have the dream I've always wanted, choosing to embrace my limitations and the Author of those limits. It's choosing to engage and be present with what's in front of me, even when my heart is stirred for places I've not yet seen and things I've not yet done.

Are you waiting for something? Don't despair. You're not alone. It's an ugly mess on this side of Heaven, but He is for us. He will make all things beautiful in their time as we seek Him in the dark.

How long did Israel wait for a Savior? How long did the world sit in the desperateness of sin and death? How long did creation yearn and mourn, groan and wail before the dawn of Jesus' birth? How much greater the chorus of hallelujah! How much more magnificent the redemption! How much better His plan than we could have ever imagined—Emmanuel, God with us.

There is this beautiful and complicated tension that seems to hold all things together. There is a tension of having received and having yet to receive. We know that Christ has come, and His kingdom continues to come, but we also know Christ is yet to return. We know that we have freedom in Christ and His Spirit in us, yet we are not sinless or free of temptation. Our bodies are still tossed about by the realities of time, age, gravity, and sickness. Our spirits are still surrounded by dark forces that pull and grab and fight us until our last and dying breath. We have not yet seen Christ face to face; we are not perfect and healed. We continue to be broken, beaten down, not destroyed—but we are still longing.

We will never not be waiting until we are with Him in eternity. We want poverty to end, hunger to cease, tears to be wiped away, and all things to be ordered and explained. Wouldn't I like to see all the frazzled and frayed ends of my life come together, woven into a beautiful tapestry? Wouldn't I like to see what soil my relentless tears have watered and what has arisen out of the dust and ashes of my cries of relief?

Oh, how we long! It is this longing that draws us to God. It is this longing, these pangs of despair that lead us back to our Creator. It is the waiting that reminds us that we are the created ones. We *must* wait because we depend on Him for all things. We *must* wait because He is the only One Who can breathe life into the dust and with the word of His mouth bring light from darkness and a beating heart from nothing. We *must* wait because none of this is about us, anyway. Waiting puts us in our place, the place where we have belonged all along, as His children.

The Night

Come to Me, all who are weary and burdened, and I will give you rest.

Matthew 11:28

Unfortunately, where once I associated night with rest, I now imagine it differently. Night is a place for arduous, relentless floundering around. I imagine the night as a land of unsettled tossing and turning under tangled sheets. It is a battlefield for me. Yet that is not what God created night to be. The night is when we are to rest. It is meant to hedge us in and hold us down, allowing us to be at peace and to heal. The night is meant for the recovery of our bodies and minds. It is meant to serve us, in the end. It is in the night that we are reminded that our work must end, our doings must cease, and it's not all up to us.

Rest is meant to envelop us. It is grace to us. I know this because in seasons without sleep, the relentlessness of life is too much. It overpowers, bears down, and grinds me to the end of myself. The night is supposed to free us from our strivings, wring out the tension from our tired muscles, and relieve us of all our stirring thoughts.

Our nights are a grace to us if we simply submit ourselves to them. We cannot sleep if we don't cease our strivings and allow rest to overtake us. Maybe, just maybe, I need to reclaim the night and remember what it was created for—it is a grace to me, instead of a hardship. The Creator of the sun is the same Author of the moon. Maybe we could remember that He is for our good after all, and He knows that we need seasons of waiting and looking to the horizon to restore us to Himself. Maybe He allows our longings to lead us to Him. What would change in me if I saw waiting as a gift to my soul instead of a battlefield?

May we trust the Author of our days as much as the Author of our nights. May we wait with renewed strength and hope, knowing we are not alone, we are not abandoned, and God is still accomplishing His work in us. He is not yet finished with us. I pray we can rest together in the dark nights of our lives, unafraid because we know He is Sovereign. Let us stay our eyes on the horizon, for the dawn has come and will come again forever.

One day, we will no longer yearn and hope for what has not come. One day, we will be gathered with Him in satiation of all our long-held dreams. One day, it will be *the* day that all our dreams come true. Be assured and reminded that as sure as the sun rises, that day will come. I hope at that time, I will meet you, and we will share together all the stories of how the King of our souls was King of our waiting and how He loved us and gave us rest through our darkest and longest nights. But in your waiting, may He give you renewed hope and satisfaction in Him, the One Who is enough, even here in your dark.

A Limited Prayer to a Limitless God

Uncontainable One, Unmeasurable One, I am humbled to think my hairs are countable, my sorrows containable, my tears collectable, my future seeable, my thoughts discernible—to think You see my every way, my every movement and thought, to think that You saw my formation, fiber upon fiber, in the hidden secret of my mother's womb.

I am altogether different from You, Who are unmeasurable in greatness, limitless in grace, unsearchable in wisdom, boundless in love for us, for me.

If the nations are dust, what am I? Do I think that I could ever thwart Your plan, Your design, Your will by my intention or accident? Do I think my sins are too great for Your limitless grace? They are finite, and You are infinite.

Oh, Sovereign, why does my endless fretting, asking, researching, and learning not rest at the feet of Your perfect plan? Meet me in my wayward ponderings, feverish petitions, and nonsensical ruminations. You are above all and in all. You see everything to come and are present there as much as right here.

Why be afraid, oh, Spirit? Your God is not limited. He crossed the heavens and came down; He conquered death and brings forth life; He can do all things seen and unseen. Could I ever bring a tree forth from a seed, a life from a womb, or make the earth quake or seas roar?

Oh, fathomless God, my limits are so many and my faith so small. Forgive me! Make my mountain of tears bring forth new life. Make the caverns of my losses become wells of new joy. Make my despair become a proclamation of praise. Gather the bits and pieces of my hopelessness and make a collage of hope. Be seen in my visible and invisible pain, as I shout out with every ounce remaining in me that You are still God and You are still good, even as I wait on You. Amen.

About the Author

Shannon Brink is a longtime nurse, soon to be nurse practitioner, from Vancouver, Canada, who has worked for many years in women's ministry and as a missionary in East Africa. She is a mother of four, wife of over fifteen years, and creative writer. You can follow her writings on shannonbrink.org, where she writes authentically about awkward spaces like waiting, loss, and suffering.

For more information about

Shannon Brink
and
Waiting is the Night
please visit:

www.shannonbrink.org

Ambassador International's mission is to magnify the Lord Jesus Christ
and promote His Gospel through the written word.

We believe through the publication of Christian literature, Jesus Christ and
His Word will be exalted, believers will be strengthened in their walk with
Him, and the lost will be directed to Jesus Christ as the only way of salvation.

For more information about
AMBASSADOR INTERNATIONAL
please visit:

www.ambassador-international.com
@AmbassadorIntl
www.facebook.com/AmbassadorIntl

Thank you for reading this book!

*You make it possible for us to fulfill our mission, and we are grateful for
your partnership.*

*To help further our mission, please consider leaving us a review on your social
media, favorite retailer's website, Goodreads or Bookbub, or our website.*

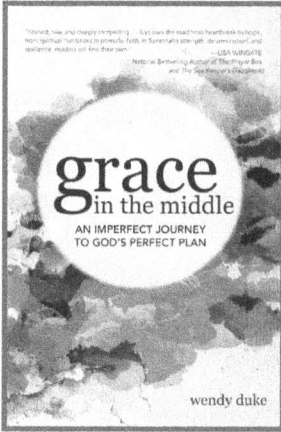

Grace in the Middle is a memoir recounting one young couple's struggle to hold on to an unraveling faith during the greatest crisis of their lives. Heartbreaking, triumphant, and funny in just the right places, this inspiring story is an authentic reflection on battling and overcoming physical illness and disability, resisting the dark doubts that plague us in the midst of tragedy, and trusting the faithfulness of God through the deep twists and turns of life.

Vanna Nguyen had escaped a war-ravaged Vietnam to make a life in America. Life seemed good and was finally settling down as Vanna planned a graduation party for her daughter Queena. But one phone call completely derailed those plans and sent Vanna and her daughters down a road that they had never dreamed they would travel. The Bloomingdale Library Attack Survivor made a name for herself, but in a way no mother would ever want. Read about two women from the same family who fought against all odds to "make beauty from ashes."

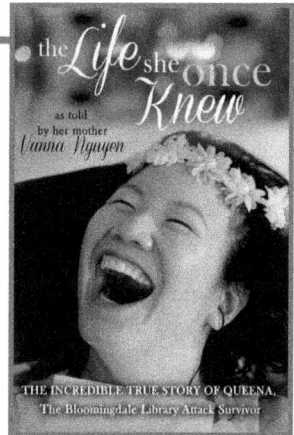

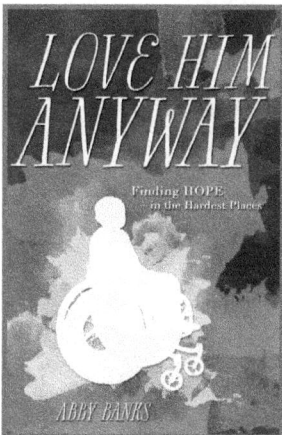

One night can change everything. Abby Banks put her healthy, happy infant son to sleep, but when she awoke the next morning, she felt as though she was living a nightmare. Her son, Wyatt, was paralyzed. In an instant, all her hopes and dreams for him were wiped away. As she struggled to come to grips with her son's devastating diagnosis and difficult rehabilitation, she found true hope in making a simple choice, a choice to love anyway—to love her son, the life she didn't plan, and the God of hope, Who is faithful even when the healing doesn't come.